# TODAY'S

# HERBAL

# HEALTH

# TODAY'S
# HERBAL
# HEALTH

FOURTH EDITION
*Revised and Updated*

## LOUISE TENNEY, M.H.

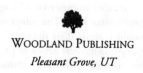

WOODLAND PUBLISHING
*Pleasant Grove, UT*

© 1997 by Woodland Publishing, Inc.
P.O. Box 160, Pleasant Grove, UT, 84062

ISBN 1-885670-06-0

Cover design by Kevn Lambson

# DEDICATION

*This book is dedicated to Josie, a dear friend who believes in herbs and who encouraged me to start this project. She was my inspiration when it looked like this book would never come about.*

# TABLE OF CONTENTS

# Introduction

*F*ourteen years ago, when I began writing the first edition of *Today's Herbal Health,* there was a remarkable lack of concise and readily available information about the herbal and natural health worlds. I am grateful this is no longer the case, that I can share with others my knowledge of natural remedies.

In my attempt to provide a complete and user-friendly text, I have organized the book into several main sections—one section provides information about single herbs, their uses and preparations; another section contains information on the many ailments that afflict the human body, along with their various natural treatments; a large portion of the book gives valuable details on the various body systems, as well as information about natural treatments used for strengthening these systems; there are also sections on diet, nutrition, and the newest nutritional products to come our way (like DHEA, melatonin, and wild yam). Finally, there is an appendix filled with everything else you might want to know about herbs. I hope this book is a useful and interesting reference that will benefit you and your family in a healthy and healing way.

# SECTION 1

# *How to Prepare Herbs*

# *Herbal Preparations*

There are a variety of ways to prepare herbs for use. The following section contains descriptions and examples of the most common types of herbal preparations, all which can be produced in your own home. To determine the best herbal preparation for your situation, you must consider the herb(s) being used and the desired results.

## BOLUS

A bolus is a suppository or internal poultice used in the rectal or vaginal area. It helps draw out toxic poisons and is the carrier for healing agents. A bolus is made by adding powdered herbs to cocoa butter, creating a thick, firm consistency. The mixture is usually placed in the refrigerator to harden and is then brought to room temperature before using. A bolus can be inserted into the rectum to treat hemorrhoids and cysts, or into the vagina to treat infections, irritations and tumors. The bolus is usually applied at night when the cocoa butter will melt with body heat, thus releasing the herbs. Herbs used in a bolus are usually astringent herbs (such as white oak bark or bayberry bark), demulcent healing herbs (such as comfrey or slipper elm), or antibiotic herbs (such as garlic, chaparral or goldenseal).

# CAPSULES

Gelatin-coated capsules are a pleasant way of taking herbs, especially when the herbs are bitter-tasting or mucilaginous. Be sure you purchase capsules from a reliable herb company This ensures the herbs will be prepared, measured and combined in the right proportion by chemists trained in herbal science. To help with swallowing and dissolving herb capsules, take them with eight ounces of pure water or herbal tea.

# COMPRESS

The effects of an herbal compress are similar to those of an ointment, with the added advantage of therapeutic heat. A compress is basically a soft pad or cloth secured on the body to provide heat, pressure or medication. It is used when herbs too strong to be taken internally need to be used for healing. Using a compress allows the herbs to be slowly absorbed in small amounts by the body. An herbal compress is used in cases of injury, contusions, and effusions. It is used for superficial ailments including swellings, pains, colds and flu. A compress always helps to stimulate circulation of blood and lymph in the body.

To prepare a compress, add one or two heaping tablespoons of the herb(s) to one cup of water and bring to a boil. Dip a sterile cotton pad, gauze or cloth into the strained liquid, drain off any excess, then place the warm compress on the affected area. It is beneficial to cover the compress with a piece of woolen material to hold in the heat. If being used on a small child, the compress should be bandaged into place. After the compress has cooled, replace it with another hot one.

A good example of an herbal compress is one made with ginger. To make a ginger compress grate two ounces of fresh ginger root and squeeze its juice into a pint of hot water until the water turns yellow. Apply the compress, having hot replacement towels ready as soon as the first one cools. A ginger compress is used to stimulate the circulation of blood and lymph, to relieve colic, to reduce internal inflammation and to restore warmth to cold joints.

# DECOCTION

To decoct means "to extract the flavor or essence of something by boiling." The term decoction is used to describe the extract obtained after boiling. An herbal decoction is similar to an infusion, but is made from the root and bark of a plant. Decoctions are used when a the root or bark is not soluble in cold or hot water, but will often yield its soluble ingredients after simmering in water for five to twenty minutes. A decoction is valuable because it contains an herb's essential mineral salts and alkaloids.

To prepare a decoction, place a teaspoon of the dried herb in an enamel or glass container with one cup of pure water. Instead of steeping the mixture, boil it—five minutes is enough if the material is finely shredded, but if the herb is hard or woody, twenty minutes is necessary to produce a good decoction. It is helpful if the plant is first soaked in cold water and then brought to a boil. Decoctions should always be strained while hot.

# EXTRACTS

An extract is a concentrated form of an herb which is obtained by mixing the herb with an appropriate solvent (such as alcohol and/or water). Herbal extracts are usually made from stimulating herbs, such as cayenne, and antispasmodic herbs, like lobelia. Extracts are rubbed into the skin as a treatment for strained muscles and ligaments, or for the relief of arthritis and other inflammations. (See Appendix for specific formulas.)

Extracts can be made by placing four ounces of dried herbs or eight ounces of fresh, bruised herbs into a jar or bottle with a tight-fitting lid. Add one pint of vinegar, alcohol or massage oil. With time, the liquid will extract the medicinal properties of the herbs. It takes about four days to get a potent extract if the herbs are powdered, and about fifteen days if the herbs are whole or cut. Your only work is to shake the bottle once or twice daily. If olive or almond oils are used in the extract, a little vitamin E can be added for a preservative. Making an extract with oil is useful if it is to be used for massage purposes. Using alcohol extract (vodka or gin) or rubbing alcohol (for external use only) allows the liquid to evaporate quickly, leaving the herbs on the skin and providing a cooling sensation.

# HYDROTHERAPY: THE HERB BATH

Hydrotherapy, the use of water for treatment of illness, is particularly popular in Europe, where health spas are quite common. But you don't have to go to a spa to enjoy their benefits! You can enjoy an herbal bath in your own home. To make a decoction for a full bath, anywhere from several ounces to a pound of plant parts should be sewn into a linen bag and boiled in a quart or more of water. The water is then added to the bath. You can also put the bag into the bath to extract more of its properties, or you can use it like a washcloth, giving yourself a healthy rubdown. Bathing with herbs accelerates their absorption through the skin. It makes them especially effective for circulation troubles, swelling of broken bones, chilblains, rheumatic diseases and gout.

# INFUSION

An infusion is an extract made from herbs with medicinal constituents in their flowers, leaves and stems. It is made by pouring hot liquid over a crude or powdered herb and allowing the mixture to steep, thus extracting the herb's active ingredients. Infusions are prepared like teas, but they are steeped longer and are considerably stronger. This method of preparation minimizes the loss of volatile elements.

The usual ratio used in preparing an infusion is about one-half to one ounce of an herb to one pint of water. Use a glass, enamel, or porcelain pot to steep the herbs for about ten to twenty minutes, then cover with a tight-fitting lid to avoid evaporation. For general purposes, strain the infusion and drink it lukewarm or cool, but to induce sweating and to break up a cold or cough, drink it hot. Remember that infusions have a short shelf life, so use them soon after you prepare them.

# OINTMENTS

Ointments are used on the skin when the active principles of herbs are needed for extended periods, as in cases of injury, contusion and effusion. Ointments stay on the skin for an extended time and allow for accelerated healing. To prepare an ointment at home, bring one or two heaping tablespoons of the herb(s) and a good helping of vaseline to a boil. (There are vaseline products made from natural sources that can be used instead of petroleum products.) The mixture then needs to be stirred and strained. After it has cooled, you can store the ointment in a jar and it will be ready for use when needed.

# OILS

When the major properties of an herb are associated with its essential oils, an oil extract will prove a useful way of preparing a concentrate. Herb oils are very useful when ointments or compresses are not practical. Oils are prepared by first macerating and pounding fresh or dried herbs. Olive oil or sesame oil is then added, two ounces of herb to one pint of oil. The mixture should then be allowed to sit in a warm place for about four days before it is used. A quicker method is to gently heat the herbs and oil in a pan for one hour. The oil can then be strained and bottled. Adding a small amount of vitamin E will help preserve the oil. Oil extracts are usually made from aromatic herbs such as eucalyptus, peppermint, spearmint and spices.

# POULTICES

An herbal poultice is a soft, moist mass of fresh, ground, or powdered herbs applied hot as a medicament to the body. A poultice is put directly on the skin to relieve inflammation, blood poisoning, venomous bites, eruptions, boils, abscesses and to promote proper cleansing and healing of the affected area. Many herbs contain ingredients necessary to draw out infections, toxins and foreign bodies embedded in the skin. Plantain and marshmallow are very good to relieve pain and muscle spasm. Cayenne is added to herbs such as lobelia, valerian, catnip and echinacea to promote stimulation and cleansing.

To prepare a poultice, moisten herbs with hot water, apple cider vinegar, herbal tea, a liniment, or a tincture. Whatever liquid you use, make sure it is hot. Cleanse the affected area with an antiseptic and then oil the skin before applying the hot poultice. A plaster is similar to a poultice. An effective plaster for drawing out fever can be made by squeezing the water out of tofu and mixing it with pastry flour and about five percent fresh ginger root. (See Appendix for other specific poultices.)

# POWDERS

Powders are simply fresh herbal agents that have been crushed into fine particles. Herbs in powder form can be taken in a capsule, in water, in herb teas, or sprinkled on food. Using powdered herbs is an ideal way to introduce herbs slowly into the diet and become adjusted to a certain dosage. For external use, powdered herbs can be mixed with oil, petroleum jelly, a little water, or aloe vera juice and applied to the skin to treat wounds, inflammation, and contusions.

# SALVES

Herbal salves are similar to ointments. A salve is made by covering fresh or dried herbs with water, bringing the mixture to a boil and letting it simmer for thirty minutes. The water is then strained off and added to an equal amount of olive oil or safflower oil. Simmer the oil/water mixture until the water has evaporated and only the oil is left. Add enough beeswax to give the mixture a salve-like consistency and pour it into a dark glass jar with a tight lid. If stored well, salves will last up to a year.

# SYRUPS

An herbal syrup is ideal for treating coughs, mucus congestion, bronchial catarrh and sore throats because it coats the area and keeps the herbs in direct contact. Syrups are especially good for children and people with sensitive palates. A syrup is made by adding about two ounces of herbs to a quart of water and gently boiling it down to one pint. While still warm, add two ounces of honey and/or glycerine. Licorice and wild cherry bark are commonly used in syrups as flavors and therapeutic agents. Other herbs used are comfrey, anise seed, fennel and Irish moss.

# TINCTURES

Tinctures are solutions of concentrated herbal extracts made with alcohol rather than water. They are more highly concentrated than infusions and decoctions, and can be kept for longer periods because alcohol is an excellent preservative. Tinctures are usually made with strong herbs that are not taken as teas. They are also useful for herbs that do not taste good or that need to be taken over an extended period of time. Tinctures are convenient for external application.

A tincture can be made by combining four ounces of powdered or cut herbs with one pint of alcohol such as vodka or brandy. Those who do not drink alcohol can make tinctures using warm (but not boiled) vinegar. Use wine or apple vinegar, but not the white variety. Allow the tincture to steep for two to four weeks, shaking every few days to encourage alcohol absorption of the herbs' medicinal properties. After four weeks, you can strain the herbs out of the liquid, but it is not necessary. Store tinctures in a cool place and keep them out of reach of children.

# SECTION 2

# *All About Herbs*

# Single Herbs

## AGRIMONY *(Agrimonia eupatoria)*

*PARTS USED: ENTIRE PLANT*

Agrimony strengthens and tones the muscles of the body because it has astringent properties which work to contract and harden tissue. Agrimony also works as a diuretic by affecting cells of the kidneys, allowing fluids to pass more readily through the kidneys. It has been recommended to help acidity and gastric ulcers because it is a good, safe stomach tonic which helps in the assimilation of food. The astringent qualities of agrimony help draw thorns and splinters from the skin. Agrimony contains vitamins B3 and K, iron and niacin.

### PRIMARY APPLICATIONS

| | |
|---|---|
| Diarrhea | Gastric disorders |
| Intestines | Jaundice |
| Kidney stones | Liver disorders |

### SECONDARY APPLICATIONS

| | |
|---|---|
| Fevers | Gallbladder |
| Hemorrhoids | Rheumatism |
| Skin diseases | Sore throat |
| Splinters | Sprains |
| Wounds, external | |

# ALFALFA *(Medicago sativa)*

## PARTS USED: LEAVES AND FLOWERS

Alfalfa helps the body assimilate protein, calcium and other nutrients. Its contents are balanced for complete absorption by the body. This herb is a body cleanser, infection fighter and natural deodorizer. It breaks down poisonous carbon dioxide and is the richest land source of trace minerals. It is a very good spring tonic, eliminates retained water, and relieves urinary and bowel problems. Alfalfa also helps in treating recuperative cases of narcotic and alcohol addiction. The enzymes in alfalfa have been known to neutralize cancer in the system.

Alfalfa contains a very rich supply of vitamins A, K, and D, as well as trace minerals. It is also high in calcium and contains phosphorus, iron, potassium and eight essential enzymes.

## PRIMARY APPLICATIONS

Anemia
Arthritis
Diabetes
Kidney cleanser
Pituitary problems

Appetite stimulant
Blood purifier
Hemorrhages
Nausea
Ulcers, peptic

## SECONDARY APPLICATIONS

Alcoholism
Appendicitis, chronic
Bowel problems
Cancer
Cramps
Diuretic (mild)
High blood pressure
Lactation
Teeth

Allergies
Body building
Bursitis
Cholesterol reducer
Digestion
Gout
Jaundice
Nosebleeds
Urinary problems

# ALOE VERA *(Aloe vera)*

*PARTS USED: LEAVES AND JUICE*

Aloe vera is known as the "first aid plant" because its antibiotic properties clean, soothe and heal. It contains compounds which promote the removal of dead skin and stimulate the normal growth of living cells. Aloe is also good for burns and wounds because it can stop pain and reduce the chance of infection and scarring while helping the healing process.

Aloe vera is a plant every household should have. It is one of the easiest plants to grow indoors and is valuable for skin irritations, minor cuts, and first and second degree thermal burns. Fresh juice from the leaves heals wounds by preventing or drawing out infections. Aloe vera also helps to heal internal tissues damaged by radiation exposure such as x-rays and radiation. This plant contains calcium, potassium, sodium, manganese, magnesium, iron, lecithin, and zinc.

## PRIMARY APPLICATIONS

Burns
Digestion
Insect bites
Scar tissue

Deodorant
Hemorrhoids
Scalds

## SECONDARY APPLICATIONS

Abrasions
Anemia
Heartburn
Poison ivy and oak
Ringworm
Sunburn
Tuberculosis
Ulcered sores

Acne
Constipation
Leg ulcers
Psoriasis
Sores
Tapeworm
Wrinkling of skin
Ulcers, peptic

# AMARANTH *(Amnaranthus spp.)*

## PARTS USED: LEAVES AND FLOWERS

Amaranth is a vitamin-packed herb that was traditionally used by Native Americans as a survival food. The mature seeds were eaten raw, mixed with corn meal, or added to soups. The leaves were used in place of spinach. Today, amaranth is used for gastroenteritis or stomach flu because it lessens irritability of the tissues. Topical application reduces tissue swelling so the herb can be used with bandages for medical treatments. A strong decoction of amaranth can be used as a vermifuge to remove worms and other parasites from the digestive tract. Amaranth is very high in iron and vitamin C. It is also high in calcium, protein and contains phosphorus, potassium, thiamine, riboflavin and niacin.

## PRIMARY APPLICATIONS

| | |
|---|---|
| Diarrhea | Dysentery |
| Menstruation, excessive | Nosebleeds |

## SECONDARY APPLICATIONS

| | |
|---|---|
| Canker sores | Gums, bleeding |
| Ulcers (stomach/mouth) | Worms |
| Wounds | |

# ANGELICA *(Angelica atripurpurea)*

## PART USED: ROOT

Angelica is very helpful for colic and digestive problems. It is considered a tonic to improve well-being and mental harmony. During the 17th and 18th centuries, the juice of the plant was used in the eyes and ears to help with dimness of sight and deafness. It has also been used for toothaches. Angelica cleans wounds and helps them to heal quickly. It is useful in all sorts of stomach and intestinal difficulties, including ulcers and vomiting with stomach cramps. It can be used for intermittent fever, nervous headaches, colic, and general weakness. Angelica contains vitamin E and calcium. Some species of this plant also contain vitamin B12, which is rare in vegetation. Diabetics should use caution with this herb because it increases sugar in the blood. It is also an emmenagogue, so it should not be used by pregnant women.

## PRIMARY APPLICATIONS

Appetite stimulant
Colds
Coughs
Gas
Rheumatism

Bronchial problems
Colic
Exhaustion
Heartburn
Tonic

## SECONDARY APPLICATIONS

Arthritis
Digestive problems
Fevers
Lung problems
Prostate problems
Stomach cramps

Backaches
Ears
Inflammation
Menstrual disorders
Sores
Toothaches

# ANISE (*Pimpinella anisum*)

## PARTS USED: OIL AND SEEDS

Anise is helpful in the removal of excess mucus from the alimentary canal. It is said by some herbalists that anise is high in estrogen, which tends to stimulate all the glands. Anise is used for loss of appetite, difficulty of digestion, and mucus obstruction associated with coughs and whooping cough. It is used as a stimulant for vital organs of the body such as heart, liver, lungs and brain. It is one of the best herbs for relieving pains for colic. Anise contains B vitamins, choline, calcium, iron, potassium and magnesium.

## PRIMARY APPLICATIONS

| | |
|---|---|
| Colic | Convulsions |
| Cough | Gas |
| Intestinal purifier | Mucus |

## SECONDARY APPLICATIONS

| | |
|---|---|
| Appetite stimulant | Breath sweetener |
| Catarrh | Colds (hard and dry) |
| Epilepsy | Nausea |
| Nervousness | Pneumonia |

# ANTLER (Deer and Elk)

## PARTS USED: ENTIRE ANTLER

Antlers are usually gathered after they have been dropped by deer or elk. Antlers have been used for thousands of years to increase vitality and longevity. They are often found in combinations and are thought to increase immunity. Antlers are rich in calcium and trace minerals important for the body.

## PRIMARY APPLICATIONS

| | |
|---|---|
| Aging | Energy |
| Hormone balance | Impotence |
| Infertility | Longevity |

## SECONDARY APPLICATIONS

| | |
|---|---|
| Anemia | Arthritis |
| Blood pressure | Fevers |
| Flu | Frigidity |
| Memory | Menopause |
| Metabolism | Miscarriage |
| Osteomyelitis | Rheumatism |
| Stress | Teeth |

# ASTRAGALUS *(Astragali membranaceus)*

## PART USED: ROOT

Astragalus has been used in traditional Chinese medicine for thousands of years. Recently, it has become popular among Western herbalists and is often found in energy tonics. It helps to increase the production of interferon, which helps stimulate and enhance the immune system. The herb is currently being reviewed by the American Cancer Society because of its positive effect on the immune system of cancer patients. Studies are also being done to find out if this herb may help to prevent viral infections such as influenza and the common cold. Astragalus has been used to treat many different ailments including chronic fatigue syndrome, pneumonia, emphysema, chronic infection, chronic cough, uterine bleeding, chronic nephritis and ulcers.

## PRIMARY APPLICATIONS

| | |
|---|---|
| Cancer | Chronic fatigue |
| Epstein-Barr syndrome | Immune system |

## SECONDARY APPLICATIONS

| | |
|---|---|
| Cysts | Edema |
| Emphysema | Nephritis |
| Pneumonia | Ulcers |

# BARBERRY *(Berberis vulgaris)*

*PART USED: BARK*

*B*arberry contains antiseptic properties which make it useful as a gargle and mouthwash. It is thought to be one of the best medicinal herb plants of the west. Barberry is used for fevers and inflammatory conditions. It influences the liver so that bile will flow more freely, which is important in almost all liver problems, especially jaundice. It also helps remove morbid matter from the stomach and bowels. It dilates the blood vessels, so is good for high blood pressure. Barberry is high in vitamin C and also contains iron, manganese, and phosphorus.

## PRIMARY APPLICATIONS

| | |
|---|---|
| Blood purifier | Diarrhea |
| Indigestion | Jaundice |
| Liver problems | Sore throat |

## SECONDARY APPLICATIONS

| | |
|---|---|
| Arthritis | Blood pressure (lowers) |
| Constipation | Dysentery |
| Dyspepsia | Fevers |
| Gallbladder | Gum diseases |
| Hemorrhages | Laxative |
| Pyorrhea | Spleen problems |
| Ulcers | |

# BARLEY *(Hordeum vulgare)*

*PART USED: JUICE (IN POWDERED FORM)*

*B*arley juice powder is produced from the juice of young barley leaves. It is essentially the same as the fresh juice and contains concentrated nutrients, live enzymes, chlorophyll, proteins, vitamins and minerals. Powdered barley juice also contains antiviral properties and is a great booster for the immune system. It has a cleansing effect on the cells, normalizes metabolism and neutralizes heavy metals like mercury. It helps to lower cholesterol and is an excellent cell detoxifier. Its high iron content helps to purify and build up the blood. It aids digestion and therefore works to strengthen the whole body. It can relieve constipation. Barley juice powder is rich in calcium, iron, magnesium, potassium, vitamin C and bioflavonoids. It also contains vitamins B1, B12 and superoxide dismutase (SOD).

### PRIMARY APPLICATIONS

| | |
|---|---|
| Anemia | Arthritis |
| Blood purifier | Boils |
| Cancer | Metal poisoning |

### SECONDARY APPLICATIONS

| | |
|---|---|
| Acne | Aids |
| Allergies | Bronchitis |
| Candida albicans | Eczema |
| Hay fever | Herpes |
| Infections | Kidney problems |
| Leprosy | Liver problems |
| Lung problems | Psoriasis |
| Skin diseases | Syphilis |
| Tuberculosis | Ulcers |

# BASIL (*Ocimum basilicum*)

## PART USED: LEAVES

Basil has been effectively used as a stimulant in cases of collapse. It also has strong antibacterial and antispasmodic properties. It is useful for whooping cough and, when applied to insect stings or venomous bites, it can help draw out poisons. Basil contains vitamins A, D, B2, calcium, phosphorus, magnesium and iron.

## PRIMARY APPLICATIONS

Bites (insect, snake)          Colds
Headaches                      Indigestion
Whooping cough

## SECONDARY APPLICATIONS

Bladder problems               Catarrh (intestinal)
Constipation                   Cramps (stomach)
Fevers                         Flu
Kidney problems                Menstruation (suppressed)
Nausea                         Nervous conditions
Respiratory infections         Rheumatism
Vomiting (excessive)           Worms

# BAYBERRY (*Myrica Cerrifera*)

## PART USED: BARK

Bayberry has long been used as a tonic, stimulating the system to help raise vitality and resistance. It can be useful in warding off colds if it is taken as soon as any symptoms appear. When taken with capsicum its healing properties are even more enhanced. Bayberry can be used as a gargle for tonsillitis and sore throat. It is also beneficial in rejuvenation of the adrenal glands, cleansing the blood stream, and washing out wastes in veins and arteries. In India, the powdered root bark of bayberry has been combined with ginger to successfully combat the deadly effects of cholera. Bayberry contains a high amount of vitamin C.

PRIMARY APPLICATIONS

| | |
|---|---|
| Cholera | Diarrhea |
| Dysentery | Glands |
| Goiter | Indigestion |
| Jaundice | Menstrual bleeding, excessive |
| Scrofula | Uterine hemorrhage |

SECONDARY APPLICATIONS

| | |
|---|---|
| Bleeding | Catarrh |
| Colitis | Dyspepsia |
| Gums, bleeding | Liver problems |
| Sluggishness | Scurvy |
| Throat, sore and ulcerated | Ulcers |
| Uterus, prolapsed | |

# BILBERRY (*Vaccinium myrtillus*)

PART USED: FRUIT

Bilberry is an old remedy that has now been rediscovered. Along with vitamin E and other supplements that supply oxygen to the blood, bilberry is considered an herb beneficial in preventing cataracts. It has the ability to protect the eyes against damage caused by diabetes. Research has found bilberry benefits the eyes because it strengthens the capillaries that surround them. This herb feeds the capillaries and improves circulation by altering the ability of fluids and nourishment to pass through them. Of course, these benefits apply to all capillaries, veins and arteries in the body, so this herb improves circulation to the feet, hands, brain, and heart. It strengthens coronary arteries, varicose veins and help in reducing the obstruction of arteries by plaque deposits. Bilberry inhibits blood platelets sticking together so blood clots can be reduced. Bilberry is rich in bioflavonoids, manganese, phosphorus, iron and zinc. It contains moderate amounts of magnesium, potassium and selenium. It contains trace amounts of calcium, sodium and silicon.

## PRIMARY APPLICATIONS

Blood vessels                     Cold hands and feet
Night blindness                   Varicose veins

## SECONDARY APPLICATIONS

Blood thinner                     Diarrhea
Dropsy                            Immune system
Kidney problems                   Light sensitive
Raynaud's disease                 Scurvy
Typhoid

# BIRCH *(Betula alba)*

## PARTS USED: BARK AND LEAVES

*B*irch contains natural properties for cleansing the blood. Dry distillation of the bark produces birch oil, which is used for certain skin complaints. Birch bark also contains a glycoside which decomposes to give methyl salicylate, a remedy for rheumatism used both in Canada and the United States. A decoction of birch leaves is recommended for baldness. A decoction can also be used as a mild sedative for insomnia. Birch powder can be used to brush teeth because it is high in natural fluoride. Birch contains vitamins A, C, E, B1 and B2. It also contains calcium, chlorine, copper, iron, magnesium, phosphorus, potassium, sodium, and silicon.

## PRIMARY APPLICATIONS

Bladder                           Blood cleanser
Eczema, external

## SECONDARY APPLICATIONS

| | |
|---|---|
| Bleeding gums | Cankers |
| Cholera | Diarrhea |
| Dysentery | Dropsy |
| Fevers | Gout |
| Kidneys | Urinary tract |

# BISTORT (*Polygonum bistorta*)

## PARTS USED: ROOT

*B*istort is one of the strongest astringents in the herb kingdom. It has antiseptic properties so is good for infectious diseases. Powdered bistort can be applied to wounds and is useful in healing all bleeding, internal and external. A decoction is used as a mouthwash and for gum problems and mouth inflammations. Bistort is also used as a wash for sores and hemorrhages. Another valuable property of the herb is that, being a member of the buckwheat family, it can be used as an emergency food. The root contains starch, and historically, in times of famine, it was dried and ground up for use as flour. Bistort contains vitamin A, vitamin B-complex and is rich in vitamin C.

## PRIMARY APPLICATIONS

| | |
|---|---|
| Bleeding, external and internal | Cholera |
| Cuts | Diarrhea |
| Dysentery | Gums |
| Hemorrhoids | Mouthwash |

## SECONDARY APPLICATIONS

| | |
|---|---|
| Bowels | Canker sores |
| Diabetes | Jaundice |
| Measles | Menstruation (regulation of) |
| Mucus | |

# BLACKBERRY *(Rubus fructicosus)*

PARTS USED: BERRIES, LEAVES AND ROOT BARK

Blackberry root tea has long been used by Native Americans as a cure for dysentery. The Chinese believe the fruit gives vigor to the whole body. When used as a tea, blackberry can dry up sinus drainage. An infusion of the unripe berries is highly esteemed for curing vomiting and loose bowels. The root contains astringent properties. The shoots of young blackberry plants are credited with fastening loose teeth in the gums. Blackberry contains vitamins A and C, iron, calcium, riboflavin, niacin and some thiamine.

### PRIMARY APPLICATIONS

| | |
|---|---|
| Bleeding | Cholera |
| Diarrhea (children) | Dysentery |
| Sinus drainage | Vomiting |

### SECONDARY APPLICATIONS

| | |
|---|---|
| Anemia | Boils |
| Eye wash | Female problems |
| Fevers | Gargle |
| Genital irritations | Gums, bleeding |
| Menstruation, excessive | Mouth irritations |
| Peristalsis, weak | Rheumatism |

# BLACK COHOSH *(Cimicigua racemosa)*

PART USED: ROOT

Black cohosh is used as a tonic for the central nervous system because it is an excellent, safe sedative. It contains natural estrogen and so helps to reduce hot flashes, contract the uterus and increase sluggish menstrual flow. The female sex hormone also helps to slow the growth of prostate tumors in men. Other healing abilities of black cohosh include loosening and expelling mucus from the bronchial tubes, neutralizing poisons in the bloodstream, and eliminating uric acid and other toxic wastes in the body. A black cohosh poultice can be used to combat all kinds of inflammation. A syrup can be used for coughs. Black cohosh contains effective amounts of calcium, potassium, magnesium, and iron. It contains some vitamin A, inositol, pantothenic acid, silicon, and phosphorus.

## PRIMARY APPLICATIONS

| | |
|---|---|
| Asthma | Bronchitis, chronic and acute |
| Epilepsy | High blood pressure |
| Hormone balance | Lungs |
| Menopause | Menstrual problems |
| St. Vitus dance | Tuberculosis |

## SECONDARY APPLICATIONS

| | |
|---|---|
| Arthritis | Bites, insect and snake |
| Childbirth | Cholera |
| Convulsions | Coughs |
| Cramps | Headaches |
| Heart stimulant | Hot flashes |
| Hysteria | Insomnia |
| Kidney problems | Liver problems |
| Lumbago | Nervous disorders |
| Rheumatism | Skin problems |
| Smallpox | Uterine problems |

# BLACK WALNUT *(Juglans nigra)*

*PARTS USED: HULLS AND LEAVES*

*B*lack walnut oxygenates the blood to kill parasites. Its extract is very useful for poison oak, ringworm and skin problems. It is also works to eliminate excessive toxins and fatty materials, and to balance sugar levels. The brown stain found in the unripe walnut husk contains organic iodine which has antiseptic healing properties. Interestingly, black walnut has also been noted to restore tooth enamel. This herb is rich in vitamin B15 and manganese. It also contains magnesium, silica, protein, calcium, phosphorus, iron and potassium.

## PRIMARY APPLICATIONS

| | |
|---|---|
| Antiseptic, external | Lactation, stops |
| Parasites, internal | Rashes, skin |
| Ringworm | Worms |

## SECONDARY APPLICATIONS

| | |
|---|---|
| Abscesses | Acne |
| Antiperspirant | Boils |
| Cancer | Carbuncles |
| Colitis | Diphtheria |
| Eczema | Eye diseases |
| Fevers | Gargle |
| Hemorrhoids | Infections |
| Liver problems | Lupus |
| Mouthsores | Poison Ivy |
| Scrofula | Tonsillitis |
| Tuberculosis | Tumors |
| Ulcers, internal | Uterus, prolapsed |
| Varicose veins | Wounds |

# BLESSED THISTLE *(Cnicus benedictus)*

## PARTS USED: *ENTIRE PLANT*

*B*lessed thistle has a long history as a tonic which helps digestion, blood circulation, and liver problems. The herb is also known to help with many female problems. Historically, the Quinault Indians steeped the whole plant to create a birth-control medicine. The herb is useful for menopausal problems and helps with cramps and hormone balance. It also works to increase mother's milk. Blessed thistle is used to fight headaches and strengthens the memory by bringing oxygen to the brain. It also has been used for treating internal cancers. The herb contains vitamin B-complex, manganese, calcium, iron, phosphorus, and potassium.

## PRIMARY APPLICATIONS

| | |
|---|---|
| Blood circulation | Blood purifier |
| Digestion | Gallbladder |
| Headaches | Heart (strengthens) |
| Hormones (balances) | Lactation |
| Liver ailments | Lungs (strengthens) |
| Menstrual problems | |

## SECONDARY APPLICATIONS

| | |
|---|---|
| Arthritis | Birth control |
| Cancer | Constipation |
| Cramps | Dropsy |
| Fevers | Gas |
| Jaundice | Kidneys |
| Leucorrhea | Memory (strengthens) |
| Respiratory infection | Senility |
| Spleen | Worms |

# BLUE COHOSH (*Caulophyllum thalictroides*)

*PART USED: ROOT*

Blue cohosh has antibacterial properties and a strong antispasmodic effect. It can relieve muscle cramps and spasms. Black cohosh helps to stretch the neck of the uterus and so eases the birthing process. The herb can help cases of slow, painful labor, but is most reliable if given some hours previous to delivery. Because of its emmenagoguic properties, it should not be used by pregnant women except during the ninth month. It is also helpful in relieving painful menstruation. Blue cohosh should be used in combination with other herbs, such as black cohosh. Blue cohosh contains vitamins E and B-complex, calcium, magnesium, phosphorus and potassium.

## PRIMARY APPLICATIONS

Cramps
Labor (induces)
Uterus (chronic problems)

Epilepsy
Nerves

## SECONDARY APPLICATIONS

Ague
Colic
Diabetes
Fits
Leucorrhea
Neuralgia
Spasms

Bladder infection
Convulsions
Dropsy
High blood pressure
Menstruation (regulation of)
Pregnancy disorders
Vaginitis

# BLUE VERVAIN *(Verbena hastata)*

*PARTS USED: ENTIRE PLANT*

*B*lue vervain is used as a natural tranquilizer. It has the ability to promote sweating and relaxation, allay fevers, settle the stomach, and produce an overall feeling of well-being. Blue vervain is one of the best herbs to help alleviate the onset of a cold, especially one involving upper respiratory inflammation. It will help expel phlegm from the throat and chest. It is also useful in menstrual problems. Blue vervain contains vitamin C, some vitamin E, calcium and manganese.

## PRIMARY APPLICATIONS

| | |
|---|---|
| Asthma | Bladder |
| Bowels | Bronchitis |
| Colds | Colon |
| Consumption | Convulsions |
| Coughs | Fevers |
| Insomnia | Stomach upset |
| Worms | |

## SECONDARY APPLICATIONS

| | |
|---|---|
| Ague | Catarrh |
| Congestion, throat and chest | Diarrhea |
| Dysentery | Earaches |
| Epilepsy | Female problems |
| Gallstones | Headaches |
| Kidney problems | Menstrual problems |
| Mucus | Nerves |
| Pneumonia | Skin diseases |
| Sores | Spleen |

# BONESET *(Eupatorium perfoliatum)*

*PARTS USED: ENTIRE PLANT*

*B*oneset is excellent as a treatment for influenza. The herb used to be called "break-bone fever" because the pain that accompanies influenza often feels like breaking bones. Dr. Shook, a noted herbalist, says that he has never known this herb to fail in overcoming the flu. Native Americans used it to reduce fever, relieve body pain and to fight colds. Boneset tea was one of the most common home remedies in the1800s. It is a mild tonic and very useful for indigestion in the elderly. Boneset contains vitamin C, calcium, magnesium, potassium and some PABA.

## PRIMARY APPLICATIONS

| | |
|---|---|
| Chills | Colds |
| Fever Prevention | Fevers (all kinds) |
| Flu | |

## SECONDARY APPLICATIONS

| | |
|---|---|
| Bronchitis | Catarrh |
| Jaundice | Liver disorders |
| Malaria | Measles |
| Mumps | Rheumatism, muscular |
| Worms | Throat (sore) |

# BORAGE *(Borago officinalis)*

*PART USED: LEAVES*

*B*orage is especially effective in healing bronchitis and soothing the digestive system. This herb has a stimulating effect on the adrenal glands kidneys. It is said to be good in restoring vitality during recovery from illness. Borage tea can be used as an eyewash for sore eyes, and it has been known to increase mother's milk. Borage contains potassium and calcium.

## PRIMARY APPLICATIONS

Bronchitis                     Catarrh (chronic)
Eyes, inflammation             Heart, strengthens
Lactation                      Rashes
Ringworm

## SECONDARY APPLICATIONS

Bladder                        Blood purifier
Colds, fever                   Digestion
Jaundice                       Insomnia preventative
Nerves (calms)                 Pleurisy

# BUCHU (*Barosma betulina*)

## PART USED: LEAVES

*B*uchu is an excellent herb for urinary organs because it absorbs excessive uric acid, thus reducing bladder irritations. In fact, buchu has a healing influence on all chronic complaints of the genitourinary tract. It is used to treat enlargement of the prostate gland and irritation of the urethra membrane. Buchu acts as a tonic, astringent and disinfectant of the mucous membranes. It is also an ingredient in some diuretics that are marketed to relieve symptoms of premenstrual bloating. Buchu is said to be useful for the first stages of diabetes.

## PRIMARY APPLICATIONS

Bladder catarrh                Kidney problems
Nephritis                      Prostate problems
Urethritis

## SECONDARY APPLICATIONS

| | |
|---|---|
| Bedwetting | Cystitis |
| Diabetes (first stages) | Dropsy |
| Gallstones | Rheumatism |
| Yeast infections | |

# BUCKTHORN *(Rhamnus frangula)*

## PARTS USED: BARK AND BERRIES

*B*uckthorn is a well-known and powerful laxative. It can have a calming effect on the gastrointestinal tract without being habit-forming. It also works on the liver and gallbladder. If taken hot, it will produce perspiration and lower fevers. An ointment made with this herb helps provide relief from itching. Bruised buckthorn leaves will stop bleeding when applied to a wound.

## PRIMARY APPLICATIONS

| | |
|---|---|
| Bleeding | Bowels |
| Constipation (chronic) | Fevers |
| Gallstones | Lead poisoning |
| Liver | |

## SECONDARY APPLICATIONS

| | |
|---|---|
| Appendicitis | Dropsy |
| Gout | Hemorrhoids |
| Parasites | Rheumatism |
| Skin diseases | Warts, external |
| Itching | |

# BUGLEWEED *(Lycopus virginicus)*

*PARTS USED: ENTIRE PLANT*

*B*ugleweed is used to relieve aches and pains. It contains compounds that contract the tissues of mucous membranes and reduce fluid discharges. Bugleweed is also used as a treatment for enlargement of the thyroid gland. Like digitalis, it works to lower the pulse, as well as equalize circulation. One of its most common uses is soothing the irritations of a cough. It is termed one of the mildest and most effective narcotics in the world.

### PRIMARY APPLICATIONS

| | |
|---|---|
| Coughs | Indigestion, nervous |
| Menstruation, excessive | Nerves |

### SECONDARY APPLICATIONS

| | |
|---|---|
| Bleeding | Colds |
| Diabetes | Diarrhea |
| Fevers | Hemorrhages, pulmonary |
| Nosebleeds | Sores |
| Tuberculosis | Ulcers |

# BURDOCK *(Arctium lappa)*

*PART USED: ROOT*

*B*urdock is an excellent blood purifier. It promotes kidney function to help clear the blood of harmful acids. It can reduce swelling around joints and help reduce calcification deposits. Burdock contains anywhere from 27 to 45 percent inulin, a form of starch, which is the source of most of its curative powers. Inulin is a substance that is important in the metabolism of carbohydrates.

When mixed with sassafras and made into a tea, this herb is said to release a strong oil that is soothing to the hypothalamus. It also aids the pituitary gland to release an ample supply of protein, which helps adjust hormone balance in the body. It is said that a poorly nourished pituitary gland is sometimes responsible for people being overweight. Burdock is rich in vitamin C and iron. It is 12 percent protein, 70 percent carbohydrate, contains some vitamin A, E, P, and B-complex, PABA, and small amounts of sulphur, silicon, copper, iodine and zinc.

## PRIMARY APPLICATIONS

| | |
|---|---|
| Arthritis | Blood purifier |
| Eczema | Gout |
| Kidney problems | Lungs |
| Rheumatism | Skin diseases |

## SECONDARY APPLICATIONS

| | |
|---|---|
| Acne | Allergies |
| Asthma | Boils |
| Bronchitis | Canker sores |
| Cancer | Dandruff |
| Fevers | Hay fever |
| Infections | Leprosy |
| Liver problems | Lumbago |
| Nervousness | Uterus, prolapsed |

# BUTCHER'S BROOM (*Ruscus aculeatus*)

## PART USED: RHIZOMES

Butcher's broom is an herb that has been used for centuries. Modern research has revealed that it has a strengthening effect on blood vessel walls. It works to constrict veins, making it effective for patients with a post-operative tendency toward circulatory problems. Other benefits of butcher's broom include improving circulation, preventing post-operative thrombosis, and preventing and healing varicose veins, phlebitis, hemorrhoids and circulatory problems. This herb increases circulation to the brain, legs and arms. It can also cause constriction of blood vessels and so is used for its anti-inflammatory properties. It will help prevent atherosclerosis and lower cholesterol levels. Because circulatory problems are one of the leading causes of death in the United States, it would be wise to consider butcher's broom.

## PRIMARY APPLICATIONS

| | |
|---|---|
| Atherosclerosis | Hemorrhoids |
| Thrombosis (blood clotting) | Varicose veins |

## SECONDARY APPLICATIONS

| | |
|---|---|
| Brain (circulation) | Circulation (increases) |
| Dropsy | Headaches |
| Jaundice | Leg cramps |
| Menstrual problems | Phlebitis (vein inflammation) |

# CALENDULA (SEE MARIGOLD)

# CAPSICUM OR CAYENNE

(*Capsicum frutescens*)
PART USED: FRUIT

Capsicum is said to be unequalled in warding off diseases. It is called a "supreme and harmless internal disinfectant." Its antibacterial properties help to relieve infectious diarrhea. Capsicum also affects circulation and increases heart action, but not blood pressure. It is said to prevent stokes and heart attacks and is used for hemorrhaging. This herb is important because its stimulating action works quickly on flu and colds.

Capsicum helps in digestion when taken with meals, and promotes normality in all secreting organs. It has the ability to rebuild tissue in the stomach and heal stomach and intestinal ulcers. Most importantly, capsicum is known as the purest and best stimulant in the herb kingdom. It is said to be a catalyst, quickly carrying all other herbs to parts of the body where they are most needed, and increasing their effectiveness. Capsicum is high in vitamins A, C, iron and calcium. It contains vitamin G, magnesium, phosphorus, and sulphur. It also has some B-complex, and is rich in potassium.

### PRIMARY APPLICATIONS

| | |
|---|---|
| Arthritis | Bleeding |
| Blood pressure equalizer | Circulation |
| Diabetes | Heart |
| High blood pressure | Kidney problems |
| Rheumatism | Strokes |
| Tumors | Ulcers |

### SECONDARY APPLICATIONS

| | |
|---|---|
| Ague | Blood cleanser |
| Bronchitis | Bruises |
| Burns | Congestion |
| Chills | Eyes |
| Fatigue | Fevers |
| Gas | Infection |
| Jaundice | Lockjaw |
| Lung problems | Mucus |
| Pancreas | Pyorrhea |
| Shock | Sprains |
| Sunburns | Throat, sore |
| Varicose veins | Wounds |

# CARAWAY *(Carum carvi)*

PART USED: SEEDS

Caraway, like anise, is a powerful antiseptic especially effective in relieving toothaches. When applied locally to the skin, it also and also acts as an anesthetic. Caraway is very useful when mixed with other herbs; for example, when used with mandrake or culver's root, it helps to correct or modify their purgative action. It is useful for all stomach problems—helps prevent fermentation in the stomach and settles the stomach after taking medicines which cause nausea. It encourages menstruation and the flow of milk, and is good for uterine cramps. It helps decrease mucus in the lungs and intestinal gas of infants. Caraway contains vitamin B-complex. It is high in calcium, potassium, and also contains smaller amounts of magnesium, lead, silicon, zinc, iodine, copper, cobalt, and iron.

## PRIMARY APPLICATIONS

| | |
|---|---|
| Appetite stimulant | Colic |
| Cramps, uterine | Digestion (acids) |
| Gas | Spasms |

## SECONDARY APPLICATIONS

| | |
|---|---|
| Colds | Female problems |
| Lactation | Mucus in lungs |
| Menstruation promoter | Stomach (settles) |
| Toothaches | |

# CASCARA SAGRADA

*(Rhaumnus purshiana)*

PART USED: BARK

C ascara sagrada is one of the best herbs available to cure chronic constipation. Cascara has this ability because its bark is rich in hormone-like oils which promote peristaltic action in the intestinal canal—they exert a remarkable action on torpor of the colon. As a result of this action, cascara is a valuable treatment for hemorrhoids due to poor bowel function. This herb helps achieve painless evacuations and, after extended usage, the bowels will function naturally and regularly from its tonic effects. It also increases secretions of the stomach, liver, and pancreas, and has been effective in helping the body rid itself of gallstones. It also has a stimulating tonic effect on all nerves it comes in contact with. Cascara sagrada contains vitamin B-complex, calcium, potassium, manganese, and traces of tin, lead, strontium and aluminum.

## PRIMARY APPLICATIONS

| | |
|---|---|
| Colon | Constipation |
| Gallbladder | Intestines |
| Liver disorders | Coughs |

## SECONDARY APPLICATIONS

| | |
|---|---|
| Croup | Digestion |
| Dyspepsia | Gallstones |
| Gout | Hemorrhoids |
| High blood pressure | Indigestion |
| Insomnia | Jaundice |
| Nerves | Pituitary |
| Spleen | Worms |

# CATNIP (*Nepeta cataria*)

## PARTS USED: WHOLE PLANT

Catnip was traditionally used by Native Americans for infant colic because it has a sedative effect on the nervous system. It is still generally used for colic, restlessness and as a pain killer. It is useful for many other ailments as well. It is effective in all cases of fevers because it helps to induce sleep and produces perspiration without increasing body heat. It is said to speedily overcome convulsions in children. It has been known to help prevent a cold if taken as a warm infusion when the first symptoms are noticed. Catnip helps with fatigue and improves circulation. It is said to help to prevent miscarriages and premature births. It also helps with the aches, pains, upset stomach and diarrhea associated with flu. Catnip is high in vitamins A, C, and B-complex. It contains magnesium, manganese, phosphorus, sodium, and has a trace of sulphur.

## PRIMARY APPLICATIONS

| | |
|---|---|
| Colds | Colic |
| Convulsions | Diarrhea |
| Digestion | Fevers |
| Flu | Gas |

## SECONDARY APPLICATIONS

| | |
|---|---|
| Anemia | Bronchitis chronic |
| Circulation (improves) | Coughs |
| Cramps, menstrual | Cramps, muscle |
| Diseases, childhood | Drug withdrawal |
| Fatigue | Headaches, nervous |
| Hemorrhoids | Hiccups |
| Infertility | Insanity |
| Lung congestion | Menstruation, suppressed |

Miscarriage (prevents)
Nicotine withdrawal
Restlessness
Skin
Spasms
Stomach upset
Worms

Morning sickness
Pain
Shock
Sores, external
Stress
Vomiting

# CAT'S CLAW (UÑA DE GATO)

*(Uncaria Tomentosa)*
PART USED: INNER BARK

Cat's claw is the name of a vine that grows on trees along the Amazon River and its surrounding foothills. It is also found in the highlands of Peru and other South American countries. Throughout the Spanish-speaking world it is well known for its medicinal value. It is also recognized as a valuable herb in Europe. Ongoing research seems to validate the usefulness of cat's claw. It is now gaining popularity in the United States as more people become familiar with the value of its multiple uses.

Cat's claw has the ability to act as an antioxidant, protecting the body from free radical damage and destroying or neutralizing carcinogens before they can damage the cells. It has been recognized that the herb helps support the body during chemotherapy and radiation, and may even inhibit the growth of cancer cells. Cat's claw has also been used successfully to treat conditions associated with a weakened immune system such as AIDS, herpes, and Epstein-Barr syndrome. Its ability to strengthen the immune function really is remarkable. Other clinical research has found that cat's claw has the ability to reduce inflammation. It has also been used to help with allergies, hemorrhoids, ulcers, parasites, Crohn's disease, and gastrointestinal disorders.

## PRIMARY APPLICATIONS

Cancer
Chemotherapy
Crohn's disease
Intestinal Problems
Irritable bowel syndrome
Parasites
Radiation
Viral Infections

Candida
Chronic fatigue syndrome
Diverticulitis
Immune system
Lupus
PMS
Ulcers

## SECONDARY APPLICATIONS

Allergies
Bursitis
Constipation
Female hormone balance

Arthritis
Colitis
Diarrhea

# CELERY (*Apium graveolens*)

## PARTS USED: ROOT, STEM AND SEEDS

Celery seeds and stems have long been used in Australia as an acid neutralizer. Celery should be cooked with milk and eaten freely to neutralize uric acid and other excess acids in the body. Such neutralization aids in the treatment of rheumatism. It also has a stimulating effect on the kidneys, producing an increased flow of urine. When taken as a tea, celery is useful for headaches. It produces perspiration and works to decrease nervousness. Celery contains vitamins A, B, C and is rich in calcium, potassium, phosphorus, sodium, and iron. It also contains smaller amounts of sulphur, silicon, and magnesium.

## PRIMARY APPLICATIONS

Arthritis
Nervousness

Lumbago
Rheumatism

## SECONDARY APPLICATIONS

Bright's disease
Diabetes
Gout
Insomnia
Neuralgia
Vomiting

Catarrah, post-nasal
Dropsy
Headaches
Liver problems
Urine retention

# CENTAURY *(Erythraea centaurium)*

## PARTS USED: ENTIRE PLANT

*C*entaury is useful during a slow convalescence because it promotes appetite and strengthens the digestive system. It also purifies the blood, regulates the gallbladder, and is an excellent tonic. This herb strengthens the bladder of the elderly and helps prevent bedwetting. It is known as a preventive in all periodic febrile diseases and helps with recovery from fevers. Centaury is good for muscular rheumatism.

## PRIMARY APPLICATIONS

Blood purifier
Fevers

Digestion promoter
Menstruation promoter

## SECONDARY APPLICATIONS

Bedwetting
High blood pressure
Jaundice
Rheumatism
Tonic
Worms

Eczema
Gallbladder
Liver
Sores, external
Ulcers
Wounds, external

# CHAMOMILE (*Anthemis nobilis*)

## PART USED: FLOWER

Chamomile is a beneficial and trustworthy herb that is worth keeping handy for emergencies. It is recognized by the orthodox medical profession as a valuable medicine for the young, especially in France and Spain. It is a soothing sedative with no harmful effects. It is useful for small babies and children who suffer from colds, stomach trouble or colitis, and helps to induce sleep. It can be used externally for eczema and inflammation. It makes a pleasant tea, good for nerves and menstrual cramps. Chamomile helps promote a natural hormone similar to thyroxine which helps rejuvenate the texture of hair and skin, and helps maintain youthful mental alertness. Chamomile has a high content of calcium and magnesium, and also contains potassium, iron, manganese, zinc and vitamin A.

## PRIMARY APPLICATIONS

| | |
|---|---|
| Appetite stimulant | Bronchitis |
| Cramps, menstrual | Fevers |
| Hysteria | Insomnia |
| Menstrual suppressant | Nervousness |

## SECONDARY APPLICATIONS

| | |
|---|---|
| Air pollution | Asthma (steam inhalant) |
| Bladder problems | Catarrh |
| Childhood diseases | Constipation |
| Colds | Coughs |
| Cramps, stomach | Diarrhea |
| Drug, withdrawal | Earache compress |
| Eye, sore | Gallstones |
| Gas | Headaches |
| Indigestion | Jaundice |
| Kidneys | Measles |

| | |
|---|---|
| Pain spasms | Stomach upset |
| Teething | Throat (gargle) |
| Tumors | Typhoid |
| Ulcers, peptic | |

# CHAPARRAL (*Larrea divaricata*)

## PARTS USED: LEAVES AND STEMS

Chaparral is a potent healer and cleanser. It has the ability to cleanse deep in muscles and tissue walls. It works on the urethral tract and lymphatic system as it tones and rebuilds tissues. Medical science believes that chaparral influences the body by inhibiting unwanted rapid growth. It is a strong antioxidant, an antitumor agent, a pain-killer, and an antiseptic. It is one of the best herbal antibiotics. Chaparral has been said to be able to take LSD residue out of the system, thereby helping eliminate recurrent flashbacks. Chaparral is high in protein, potassium, and sodium. It also contains silicon, tin, aluminum, sulphur, chlorine, and barium.

## PRIMARY APPLICATIONS

| | |
|---|---|
| Arthritis | Blood purifier |
| Cancer | Leukemia |
| Tumors | |

## SECONDARY APPLICATIONS

| | |
|---|---|
| Aches | Acne |
| Allergies | Backaches, chronic |
| Boils | Bowels |
| Bruises | Bursitis |
| Cataracts | Colds |
| Cuts and wounds | Eczema |
| Eyes (strengthens) | Hemorrhoids |

Kidney infection
Psoriasis
Rheumatism
Uterus, prolapsed

Prostate
Respiratory system
Stomach disorders
Venereal diseases

# CHICKWEED (*Stellaria media*)

PARTS USED: ENTIRE PLANT

*C*hickweed is valuable for treating blood toxicity, fevers, and inflammation. Its mucilage elements are known to help stomach ulcers and inflamed bowels. Chickweed will help dissolve plaque in blood vessels as well as other fatty substances in the body. It acts as an antibiotic in the blood, and has been called an effective anticancer agent. Chickweed can be used in poultice form for boils, burns, skin diseases, sore eyes and swollen testes. It is a mild herb and has been used as a food as well as medicine. Chickweed is rich in iron, copper and vitamin C. It also contains calcium, sodium, vitamins D and B-complex, some manganese, phosphorus, and zinc.

## PRIMARY APPLICATIONS

Appetite depressant
Blood purifier
Obesity
Ulcers

Bleeding
Convulsions
Skin rashes

## SECONDARY APPLICATIONS

Arteriosclerosis
Blood poisoning
Bruises
Cancer preventive
Constipation
Eye infections

Asthma
Bronchitis
Bursitis
Colitis
Cramps
Gas

Hemorrhoids
Mucus
Testicles (swollen)
Water retention

Lung congestion
Pleurisy
Tissues (inflamed)
Wounds

# CHICORY *(Cichorium intybus)*

*PARTS USED: FLOWERING PLANT AND ROOT*

Chicory was well known in ancient Rome as a food and blood purifier. It has many of the same constituents as dandelion. Chicory tea helps eliminate unwanted phlegm from the stomach and is good for an upset stomach. Regular use of the tea is also recommended for gallstones. Chicory is good for conditions caused by excess uric acid, such as gout, rheumatics and joint stiffness. It has also been used as a wash for boils and sores. The sap of the stems is used for poison ivy and sunburned skin. Chicory is rich in vitamins A, C, G, B, K, and P.

## PRIMARY APPLICATIONS

Blood purifier
Jaundice
Phlegm (expels)

Calcium deposits
Liver problems

## SECONDARY APPLICATIONS

Anemia
Arthritis
Digestion
Gout
Infertility
Kidney problems
Rheumatism
Tonic

Arteriosclerosis
Congestion
Gallstones
Glands
Inflammations
Poultice
Spleen problems

# CHINCHONA *(Cinchona calisaya)*

PART USED: BARK

*C*hinchona contains quinine, an alkaloid which suppresses cell enzymes and acts as a disinfectant in cases of malaria and rheumatism. It is also an effective preventative for influenza. It is one of the best tonics used for all febrile and typhoid conditions. It strengthens the stomach during convalescence and works on the entire central nervous system. The liquid extract has even been used as a cure for drunkenness.

PRIMARY APPLICATIONS

| | |
|---|---|
| Fevers, intermittent | Malaria |
| Jaundice | Parasites |

SECONDARY APPLICATIONS

| | |
|---|---|
| Dropsy | Flu |
| Heart palpitations | Hysteria |
| Influenza preventative | Menstrual problems |
| Measles | Nervous disorders |
| Rheumatism | Scrofula |
| Smallpox | Typhoid fever |

# CLOVES *(Eugenia caryophyllata)*

PART USED: SEEDS

*C*loves contain one of the most powerful germicidal agents in the herb kingdom. A few drops of clove oil in water will stop vomiting and clove tea with relieve nausea. The oil of cloves is also a diffusive stimulant. It can be used to relieve a toothache when dropped into a cavity, and is frequently used as a remedy for bad breath. Cloves increase circulation of the blood and promote digestion. Cloves contain vitamins A, B-complex, C, potassium, phosphorus, calcium, magnesium and sodium.

## PRIMARY APPLICATIONS

| | |
|---|---|
| Bad breath | Bronchial catarrh |
| Circulation, poor | Dizziness |
| Earache | Nausea |

## SECONDARY APPLICATIONS

| | |
|---|---|
| Blood pressure, low | Colitis (mucus) |
| Diarrhea | Dysentery |
| Epilepsy | Gas |
| Indigestion | Pain |
| Palsy | Spasms |
| Toothache | Vomiting |
| Sexual stimulant | |

# COLTSFOOT (Tussilago farfara)

## PARTS USED: FLOWERS AND LEAVES

Coltsfoot is known as a remedy for coughs and other respiratory ailments. The ingredients of its flowers are chiefly expectorant in effect and very soothing to the mucous membranes. Coltsfoot has a calming effect on the throat, as well as on the brain's cough-activating mechanism. This explains why, when used in tea form with horehound and marshmallow, it is one of nature's best cough remedies. Coltsfoot contains a high percentage of mucilage and saponins which have disinfectant and anti-inflammatory effects that ease respiratory problems. The herb is rich in vitamins A and C, and also contains calcium, zinc, potassium, vitamins P, B12, and B6. It also has traces of iron, manganese, and copper.

## PRIMARY APPLICATIONS

| | |
|---|---|
| Asthma | Bronchitis |
| Catarrah | Coughs |
| Lung problems | Mucus |

## SECONDARY APPLICATIONS

| | |
|---|---|
| Chills | Colds |
| Diarrhea | Emphysema |
| Hoarseness | Inflammation |
| Pleurisy | Pneumonia |
| Swellings | Tracheitis (calms) |
| Tuberculosis | |

# COMFREY (Symphytum officinale)

## PARTS USED: LEAVES AND ROOTS

Comfrey is one of the most valuable herbs known to botanic medicine. It has been used with success for centuries as a wound-healer and bone-knitter. It feeds the pituitary with its natural hormone and helps strengthen the body skeleton. It helps in the calcium/phosphorus balance by promoting strong bones and healthy skin. It helps promote the secretion of pepsin and is a general aid to digestion. It generally has a beneficial effect on all parts of the body. It is one of the finest healers of the respiratory system, and can be used both internally and externally for healing of fractures, wounds, sores and ulcers. It has been used with great success to check hemorrhage, whether from the stomach, lungs, bowels, kidneys or piles. Comfrey is rich in vitamins A and C. It is high in calcium potassium, phosphorus, and protein. It contains iron, magnesium, sulphur, copper and zinc, as well as eighteen amino acids. It is a good source of the amino acid hysine, usually lacking in diets that contain no animal products.

## PRIMARY APPLICATIONS

| | |
|---|---|
| Anemia | Arthritis |
| Blood cleanser | Broken bones |
| Boils and sores | Bruises |
| Burns | Emphysema |
| Fractures | Lungs |
| Swelling | Sprains |

## SECONDARY APPLICATIONS

| | |
|---|---|
| Allergies | Asthma |
| Bladder | Bleeding |
| Bronchitis | Bursitis |
| Cancer | Colds |
| Colitis | Coughs |
| Cramps | Diarrhea |
| Digestion | Eczema |
| Fatigue | Gangrene |
| Gout | Hay fever |
| Infections | Insect bites |
| Kidney stones | Leg cramps |
| Pain | Pleurisy |
| Pneumonia | Respiratory problems |
| Sinusitis | Skin trouble |
| Stomach trouble | Tonic |

# CORNFLOWER (CYANI)

*(Centaurea cyanus)*
PARTS USED: ENTIRE PLANT

Cornflower was used by the Plains Indians as an antidote for snakebites, insect bites and stings. Its nervine powers are highly rated by herbalists. The water distilled from cornflower petals has been used as a remedy for weak eyes. The dried powder can be used on bruises. Taken in wine, the seeds, leaves or distilled water of the herb are very good against infectious diseases. Cornflower is good for ulcers and sores in the mouth. It is also used as a remedy in certain forms of temporary paralysis. This herb has properties similar to those of blessed thistle.

PRIMARY APPLICATIONS

Conjunctivitis
Diseases
Nervous disorders

Corneal ulcers
Eye disorders
Poisonous bites and stings

SECONDARY APPLICATIONS

Dermatitis
Indigestion, chronic
Mumps
Toothache

Fevers, pestilential
Infection
Sight (weak)

# CORNSILK *(Stigmata maidis)*

PART USED: SILK

Cornsilk is used for bladder complaints because it has a cleansing effect on urea as it circulates. It is also valuable in the treatment of renal and cystic inflammations, and works on morbid deposits with its antiseptic powers. Physicians have used cornsilk as a diuretic and for conditions of cystitis. This herb is rich in vitamin K. It also contains vitamin B, PABA, and silicon.

PRIMARY APPLICATIONS

Bladder problems
Kidney problems

Heart trouble

SECONDARY APPLICATIONS

Arteriosclerosis
Cholesterol

Bedwetting
Cystic irritation

Gonorrhea
Obesity
Urinary problems

High blood pressure
Prostate

# COUCH GRASS *(Agropyron repens)*

*PARTS USED: ENTIRE PLANT*

Couch grass is well known for its beneficial effects on the urinary system. It is especially used for cystitis and the treatment of catarrhal diseases of the bladder. It has been known to help eliminate stones and gravel from the kidneys and bladder. Couch grass extracts are known to have antibiotic effects against a variety of bacteria and molds. Couch grass is rich in vitamins A, C, and B-complex. It is high in silicon, potassium, and sodium, and contains smaller amounts of magnesium and calcium.

## PRIMARY APPLICATIONS

Bladder infections
Catarrhal conditions
Jaundice
Rheumatism

Blood purifier
Cystitis
Kidney problems
Urinary Infections

## SECONDARY APPLICATIONS

Bright's disease
Constipation
Female disorders
Gout
Lumbago
Prostate glands

Bronchitis
Eyes (strengthens)
Fevers
Gravel
Lungs
Skin diseases

# CRAMP BARK *(Viburnum opulus)*

*PARTS USED: BARK AND BERRIES*

Cramp bark is considered a very valuable herb because it is one of the best female regulators in nature. It has been recommended to help with pregnancy, after-pains, cramps, and especially the nervous discomforts of pregnancy. It is recognized as a uterine sedative and an antispasmodic. In Russia, the berries (fresh or dried) are used for high blood pressure, heart problems, coughs, colds, lungs, kidneys, and bleeding ulcers. Externally, a decoction of flowers has been used for eczema and other skin conditions. Cramp bark contains potassium, calcium and magnesium. The plant's berries are sometimes used like cranberries. They are very rich in vitamins C and K.

## PRIMARY APPLICATIONS

| | |
|---|---|
| Asthma | Convulsions |
| Cramps | Heart palpitation |
| Hypertension | Hysteria |
| Leg cramps | Nervousness |
| Spasms | Urinary problems |

## SECONDARY APPLICATIONS

| | |
|---|---|
| Colic | Constipation |
| Dysentery | Epilepsy |
| Fainting | Fits |
| Gallstones | Gas |
| Jaundice | Lockjaw |
| Miscarriage | Neuralgia |
| Ovarian irritations | Pregnancy (after-pains) |
| Pulse (regulates) | Rheumatism |

# CRANBERRY *(Vaccinium macrocarpon)*

PART USED: FRUIT

Cranberry is a very small fruit, but its size is deceptive—the little red berry has great nutritional value. Cranberries have long been known for their healing properties. During the 1800s, American sailors stored cranberries on their ships and ate them to prevent scurvy. The fruit and its juice are mainly used to treat bladder infections and urinary tract infections. Studies have found beneficial results with women suffering from recurrent urinary tract problems. The primary bacteria associated with urinary tract infections is *E. coli*, which prefers an alkaline environment to grow. Studies have found that certain properties of cranberries make urine more acidic and this reduces the likelihood of bacteria adhering to the lining of the urinary tract. The usual course of action when treating urinary infections is antibiotics. This treatment is often not productive, especially for those individuals who suffer from recurrent infections. Antibiotics may solve the problem temporarily, but they can cause other difficulties, such as vaginal yeast infections. The cranberry cure seems to be more effective. Cranberries are rich in iron, potassium, vitamins B and C.

PRIMARY APPLICATIONS

Bladder infections
Urinary tract infections

Kidney problems

SECONDARY APPLICATIONS

Bedwetting
Colds

Bladder problems

# CULVER'S ROOT *(Varoniscastrum virgincum)*

*PART USED: ROOT*

Culver's root has a gentle relaxing effect on the liver. It is also considered a tonic for the stomach. It helps with intestinal indigestion, purifies the blood, and removes catarrhal obstructions and congestions in a mild, natural way. Culver's root should be taken with an herb that helps expel gas (such as fennel). Its action is similar to mandrake, but concentrates more on the duodenum. Culver's root contains potassium and magnesium.

### PRIMARY APPLICATIONS

| | |
|---|---|
| Blood purifier | Diarrhea |
| Liver problems | Stomach problems |

### SECONDARY APPLICATIONS

| | |
|---|---|
| Fevers | Food poisoning |
| Syphilitic diseases | |

# DAMIANA *(Turnera aphrodisiaca)*

*PART USED: LEAVES*

Damiana has stimulating properties and is traditionally used for nervousness, weakness and exhaustion. It is one of the safest and most popular herbs claimed to restore natural sexual capacities and functions. This herb has been recommended for increasing sperm count in males, and strengthening the egg in females. It helps to achieve hormonal balance in women, and, in Mexico, is used for female disorders. It is useful for increasing sexual prowess in persons who suffer from sexual debility. Damiana is good for renewing and revitalizing anyone in a state of physical exhaustion.

## PRIMARY APPLICATIONS

| | |
|---|---|
| Bronchitis | Emphysema |
| Hormone balancer | Hot flashes |
| Menopause | Parkinson's disease |
| Sexual stimulant | |

## SECONDARY APPLICATIONS

| | |
|---|---|
| Brain tonic | Energy/Exhaustion |
| Female problems | Frigidity |
| Nervousness | Prostate |

# DANDELION (*Taraxacum officinale*)

## PARTS USED: LEAVES AND ROOT

**D**andelion benefits the liver. It has the ability to clear obstructions and stimulate the liver to detoxify poisons. It should be also considered a valuable survival food. It contains all the nutritive salts that are required by the body to purify the blood. Dandelion promotes a healthy circulation, strengthens weak arteries, cleanses skin blemishes and restores the gastric balance in patients who have suffered from severe vomiting.

The juice of the broken stem can be used for warts. It should be applied and then allowed to dry. If used daily for two or three days, the wart will dry up. Dandelion is also useful for corns, acne and blisters. A diet which includes dandelion greens will improve the tooth enamel. This herb is a natural source of protein. It is rich in vitamins A B, C and E. It is an excellent source of potassium, calcium and sodium. It contains some phosphorus, iron, nickel, cobalt, tin, copper, and zinc.

## PRIMARY APPLICATIONS

| | |
|---|---|
| Anemia | Blisters, external |
| Blood pressure (lowers) | Blood purifier |

Endurance

Gallbladder

Liver problems

## SECONDARY APPLICATIONS

| | |
|---|---|
| Age spots | Constipation |
| Corns | Cramps |
| Dermatitis | Diabetes |
| Eczema | Fatigue |
| Fever | Gout |
| Jaundice | Hypoglycemia |
| Metabolism (stimulates) | Psoriasis |
| Rheumatism | Spleen |
| Stomach | Warts |

# DEVIL'S CLAW

*(Harpagophytum procumbens)*
PART USED: ROOT

*D*evil's claw has been proven to positively affect arthritis, rheumatism, diabetes, arteriosclerosis, and liver, kidney and bladder diseases. Experiments have shown that regular use of a decoction of devil's claw will help hardened vascular walls to once again become elastic. It also helps produce a generalized feeling of strength, which seems to improve the complaints of old age. Devil's claw has properties similar to chaparral in that it has natural cleansing agents which clear the body of toxic impurities. It has been suggested that a healthy person should use devil's claw once a year to cleanse the most important body systems, lymph and blood.

## PRIMARY APPLICATIONS

| | |
|---|---|
| Arteriosclerosis | Arthritis |
| Bladder (strengthens) | Blood purifier |

Cholesterol
Kidneys (strengthens)
Pollution (air)
Stomach problems

Diabetes
Liver diseases
Rheumatism

## SECONDARY APPLICATIONS

Gallstones
Malaria

Gout

# DONG QUAI *(Angelica sinensis)*

### PART USED: ROOT

Dong quai is known as the queen of female herbs. It has been claimed to be very effective against almost every type of complaint dealing with the female system. It possesses constituents for nourishing female glands and strengthening all internal body organs and muscles. It also helps to rebuild the blood and improve the condition of a pregnant woman. Dong quai has a tranquilizing effect on the central nervous system and gives nourishment to the brain cells. It nourishes the blood, lubricates the intestines, and promotes growth of the womb. It is useful in aiding recovery from an accident if internal bleeding and body bruises exist. Dong quai contains vitamins A, B12, and E.

## PRIMARY APPLICATIONS

Anemia
Blood purifier
Female glands
Menopause

Bleeding, internal
Brain nourisher
Hot flashes
Menstruation (regulator)

## SECONDARY APPLICATIONS

Abdominal ache
Angina

Aches
Bruises

Chills
Clots (blood)
Cramps
Hypertension
Lumbago
Stomach

Circulation
Constipation
Headaches, migraine
Hypoglycemia
Metabolism
Tumors

# ECHINACEA (*Echinacea augustifolia*)

PART USED: ROOT

*E*chinacea stimulates the immune response, increasing the production of white blood cells and thus improving the body's ability to resist infections. In essence, it is a natural antibiotic. It improves lymphatic filtration and drainage, and helps remove toxins from the blood. It is considered a nontoxic way of cleansing the body. Echinacea is said to be good for enlarged or weak prostate glands. It has also been used with chickweed to help in weight loss. Echinacea contains vitamins A, E, and C, iron, iodine, copper, sulphur and potassium.

## PRIMARY APPLICATIONS

Blood builder
Blood poisoning
Boils
Infections (prevents)
Prostate problems

Blood diseases
Blood purifier
Infections, external
Lymph glands

## SECONDARY APPLICATIONS

Acne
Bites, poisonous
Carbuncle
Eczema
Gangrene
Gonorrhea

Antiseptic
Cancer
Diphtheria
Fevers
Glands, swollen
Gums

Hydrophobia
Leukemia
Peritonitis
Strep throat
Typhoid fever

Indigestion
Mucus
Sores, infected
Syphilis
Tonsillitis

# ELDERFLOWER (Sambucus nigra)

*PARTS USED: FLOWERS AND BERRIES*

Elderflower is considered one of most versatile herbs for treating disease. It is able to detoxify body cells, increase blood circulation and promote sweating. It is an alterative, blood purifier and cell cleanser. Elderflower contains constituents that act as sedatives and relieve pain. It works as an expectorant and an anti-inflammatory agent. An elderflower and peppermint blend will combat colds, flu and fevers. Elderflower is an excellent remedy for fevers when combined with goldenseal and yarrow. For lung congestion or asthma, this herb works will when combined with mullein. Elderflower contains vitamins A, C, and bioflavonoids.

## PRIMARY APPLICATIONS

Allergies
Bronchitis
Fevers
Pneumonia

Asthma
Colds
Hay fever
Sinus congestion

## SECONDARY APPLICATIONS

Brain inflammation
Digestive problems
Eye infections
Gas
Joints, swollen
Skin diseases

Cancer
Ear infections
Flu
Hemorrhoid
Nerves
Ulcers

# ELECAMPANE (*Inula helenium*)

*PART USED: ROOT*

*E*lecampane is one of the richest sources of natural insulin, and is therefore helpful for the pancreas. It gives relief from respiratory difficulties and assists expectoration. It has antiseptic properties and is used in Spain as a surgical dressing. Elecampane has been used to combat intestinal worms, reduce water retention, lessen tooth decay, and firm the gums. It is usually preferred in combination with other herbs. Elecampane contains calcium, potassium and sodium.

## PRIMARY APPLICATIONS

Bronchitis, chronic          Coughs

## SECONDARY APPLICATIONS

Asthma                          Bladder catarrh
Colic                           Convulsions
Cramps                          Digestion
Disposition (helper)            Female problems
Lungs                           Menstrual problems
Phlegm (expels)                 Poison, counteracts
Stomach tonic                   Urethra (catarrhal)
Whooping cough                  Worms

# EPHEDRA (*Ephedra species*)

*PARTS USED: ENTIRE PLANT*

*E*phedra is closely related to adrenaline and has some of the same properties. It stimulates the nervous system and acts directly on the muscle cells. This herb contains substances that effect all blood vessels, especially the small arteries and capillaries.

It helps the heart to have a slower and stronger beat. Ephedra is also used in Europe for treating rheumatism and syphilis. The juice of the ephedra berry has been noted to reduce respiratory problems. It is considered a bronchial dilator and decongestant. Ephedra contains some vitamin B12, cobalt, strontium, nickel, and copper.

### PRIMARY APPLICATIONS

| | |
|---|---|
| Blood purifier | Bronchitis |
| Bursitis | Headaches |
| Kidneys | Venereal disease |

### SECONDARY APPLICATIONS

| | |
|---|---|
| Arthritis | Asthma |
| Bleeding, internal | Blood pressure (normalizes) |
| Colds | Depression |
| Diphtheria | Drug overdose |
| Fever | Gallbladder |
| Hayfever | Heart palpitations |
| Joint problems | Menstruation |
| Muscle problems | Nosebleeds |
| Pain | Pneumonia |
| Sinus | Skin diseases |

# EUCALYPTUS (*Eucalyptus globulus*)

### PART USED: OIL

*E*ucalyptus has potent antiseptic properties. Oil extracted from the leaves works to prevent infections and is helpful against poisonous germs. Eucalyptus oil has various other abilities—it can be sniffed to clear sinus congestion, mixed with water to make a good insect repellent, and a small drop on the tongue will help nausea. Eucalyptus could be generally described as a life-giver, purifier, vitalizer, and sweetener of all organic matter. Another interesting property of eucalytpus is that its leaves convert oxygen into ozone.

### PRIMARY APPLICATIONS

| | |
|---|---|
| Bronchitis | Lungs |
| Neuralgia | Sores, external |

### SECONDARY APPLICATIONS

| | |
|---|---|
| Asthma | Boils, external |
| Burns | Cancer |
| Carbuncles, external | Catarrh |
| Croup | Diphtheria |
| Fever | Indigestion |
| Malarial diseases | Nausea |
| Paralysis | Pyorrhea |
| Throat, sore | Typhoid |
| Ulcers, external | Uterus, prolapsed |
| Worms | Wounds |

# EVENING PRIMROSE

(*Oenothera biennis*)
PARTS USED: *BARK, LEAVES, OIL*

*E*vening primrose stimulates the liver, spleen and digestive apparatus. It reduces alimentary toxins that result from a faulty diet and adversely affect the central nervous system. Evening primrose slows down the speed at which cholesterol is made by the body, and has been found effective in lowering cholesterol levels, inhibiting the formation of clots, and lowering the blood pressure of people with mild to moderate hypertension. It also opens up blood vessels and relieves the pain of angina. Evening primrose oil prevents inflammation and controls arthritis. It has been used in

Europe to treat multiple sclerosis. Evening primrose contains minerals and is high in potassium and magnesium. It is also a good source of prostaglandins, hormone-like substances necessary for health.

## PRIMARY APPLICATIONS

Cardiovascular health               High blood pressure
Nerves                              Obesity
Prostate                            Skin disorders
Rheumatoid Arthritis

## SECONDARY APPLICATIONS

Alcoholism                          Allergies
Bowel problems                      Cancer
Colds                               Cramps, menstrual
Female disorders                    Glaucoma
Headaches, migraine                 Hyperactivity (in children)
Mental depression                   Multiple sclerosis
Neuralgia                           Obesity
Sedative effect                     Skin irritation
Ulcers

# EYEBRIGHT (*Euphrasia officinalis*)

## PARTS USED: ENTIRE PLANT

*E*yebright aids in stimulating the liver to clean the blood and relieve the conditions that effect the clarity of vision and thought. It is useful for inflammations because of its cooling and detoxifying properties. It has antiseptic properties that fight infections of the eyes. It has traditionally been used as a remedy for eye problems such as failing vision, eye inflammation and ulcers, conjunctivitis, and even eye strain. Eyebright will strengthen all parts of the eye and provide an elasticity to the nerves and optic devices responsible for sight. It is extremely rich in vitamins A and C. It also contains vitamins B-complex, D, and E, iron, silicon, and a trace of iodine, copper, and zinc.

## PRIMARY APPLICATIONS

Blood cleanser
Colds
Liver stimulant

Cataracts
Eye disorders and infections

## SECONDARY APPLICATIONS

Black-eye compress
Coughs
Hayfever
Head colds
Memory
Styes (dissolves)

Congestion
Earache
Headaches and colds
Hoarseness
Sinus congestion

# FALSE UNICORN (Chamaelirium luteum)

PART USED: ROOT

*F*alse unicorn is an excellent overall tonic. It contains strong turpentine constituents and antiseptic principles. It is useful to the mucous membranes and good for a delicate stomach. It has been said that it is as good as pumpkin seeds for the removal of tapeworms. False unicorn also stimulates and corrects problems of the reproductive organs in men and women. It is important for menopausal problems because it affects uterine disorders, headaches and depression. False unicorn is high in vitamin C. It also contains copper, sulphur, cadmium, cobalt, molybdenum, and traces of zinc.

## PRIMARY APPLICATIONS

| | |
|---|---|
| Colic | Coughs |
| Digestive problems | Kidneys |
| Miscarriage (prevents) | Prostate |

## SECONDARY APPLICATIONS

| | |
|---|---|
| Appetite stimulant | Bright's disease |
| Depression | Diabetes |
| Enuresis | Gastrointestinal weaknesses |
| Headaches | Menopause |
| Nausea | Ovaries |
| Uterine problems | |

# FENNEL (*Foeniculum valgare*)

## PART USED: SEEDS

*F*ennel helps to take away the appetite. It improves digestion, has a diuretic effect, and works to move waste material out of the body. It also helps to stabilize the nervous system and is recommended as a sedative for small children. Because it influences nerves, fennel works well as an anticonvulsive and pain-reliever. It is also helpful in cases of persistent cough and bronchitis. When boiled with barley, it aids lactation. Fennel contains potassium, sulphur and sodium.

## PRIMARY APPLICATIONS

| | |
|---|---|
| Colic | Intestinal problems |
| Sedative for children | |

## SECONDARY APPLICATIONS

| | |
|---|---|
| Appetite depressant | Bronchitis |
| Congestion | Convulsions |
| Coughs | Cramps, abdominal |

Digestive aid
Gas
Lactation (promotes)

Female problems
Gout
Nervous disorders

# FENUGREEK *(Trigonella foenum-graecum)*

## PART USED: SEEDS

*F*enugreek has the ability to soften and dissolve hardened masses of accumulated mucus. It expels mucus and phlegm from the bronchial tubes. It also helps to expel toxic waste through the lymphatic system. It has antiseptic properties and kills infections in the lungs. Fenugreek contains lecithin, which dissolves cholesterol, and lipotropic substances, which dissolve deposits of fat and prevent fatty accumulations and water retention. Fenugreek used with lemon juice and honey soothes and nourishes the body and helps to reduce fevers. It is rich in vitamins A and D, minerals and protein. It also contains an oil that resembles cod liver oil, vitamins B1, B2 and B3, choline, lecithin, and iron.

## PRIMARY APPLICATIONS

Bronchial catarrh
Lung infections
Stomach irritations

Cholesterol (dissolves)
Mucus (dissolves)

## SECONDARY APPLICATIONS

Abscess
Blood poisoning
Body odor
Fevers (reduce)
Lactation
Ulcers
Water retention

Bad breath
Boils
Carbuncles
Inflammations
Throat gargle
Uterus
Wounds (poultice)

# FEVERFEW *(Chrysanthemum parthenium)*

## PARTS USED: LEAVES AND FLOWERS

*F*everfew has long been used as a natural remedy for pain relief and is considered an excellent remedy for severe headaches. In times past, feverfew was used just as aspirin and codeine are used today. The herb was used to treat any ailment where chills, fever and headache developed. Today, feverfew is also known to be effective on migraine headaches. It is good for relieving colds, dizziness, tinnitus, and inflammation from arthritis. Feverfew contains elements that work synergistically to regulate normal function of the body. It works gradually and with a gentle action that allows the body to heal itself. Feverfew contains high amounts of iron, niacin, manganese, phosphorus, potassium, and selenium. It also contains vitamins A and C, silicon, sodium and zinc.

## PRIMARY APPLICATIONS

| | |
|---|---|
| Chills | Colds |
| Fever | Headaches |
| Inflammation | Migraine headaches |
| Sinus headaches | |

## SECONDARY APPLICATIONS

| | |
|---|---|
| Aches | Ague |
| Allergies | Arthritis |
| Circulation | Digestion |
| Dizziness | Female problems |
| Hot flashes | Insect bites (external) |
| Menopause symptoms | Menstruation (promotes) |
| Nervous headaches | Nervous hysteria |
| Tinnitus | Vertigo |

# FIGWORT (Scrophularia nodosa)

PARTS USED: LEAVES, STEMS AND ROOTS

*F*igwort is essentially a skin medication used for eczema, scabies, tumors and rashes. But it also provides hormone-like materials that help soothe the digestive organs and clean the kidneys. It is a diuretic as well as an efficient pain killer when nothing stronger is at hand. In Wales, this herb is used to treat circulatory disorders and is especially good at reducing varicose veins. Figwort can be used as a poultice for ulcers, piles, scrofulous glands in the neck, sores, wounds and toothaches.

## PRIMARY APPLICATIONS

| | |
|---|---|
| Abrasions | Athlete's foot |
| Cradle cap | Fever |
| Impetigo | Restlessness |
| Skin diseases | Tumors (skin) |

## SECONDARY APPLICATIONS

| | |
|---|---|
| Anxiety | Burns |
| Cuts | Digestive organs |
| Eczema | Hemorrhoids |
| Insomnia | Kidneys |
| Menstrual flow (increases) | Nightmares |
| Worms | |

# FLAXSEED (Linum usitatissimum)

PART USED: SEEDS

*F*laxseed is one of the richest natural sources of essential fatty acids. For that reason alone it is of great worth. It is also a natural laxative. It soothes and provides mucilaginous roughage. It heals the body as it nourishes. Flaxseed has also been used for sickly babies because it enriches the blood and strengthens the nerves. It can be used as a poultice or compress, but needs to be applied as hot as one can stand it. Flaxseed contains essential fatty acids, calcium and potassium.

### PRIMARY APPLICATION

| | |
|---|---|
| Arthritis | Cardiovascualar health |
| Autoimmune diseases | Constipation |
| Cholesterol levels, lowers | Skin disorders |

### SECONDARY APPLICATIONS

| | |
|---|---|
| Bronchitis | Colds |
| Gallstones | Heart (strengthens) |
| Jaundice | Liver complaint |
| Lung problems | Pleurisy |
| Pneumonia | Rheumatism, muscular |

# GARCINIA (Garcinia cambogia)

### PART USED: FRUIT

Garcinia has been found to be beneficial in curbing the appetite, thus aiding weight control. This herb contains more than 50 percent hydroxycitric acid which is known to block the formation of fatty tissue. Garcinia helps in slowing the storage of fats in the body and in burning fat (thermogenesis).

### PRIMARY APPLICATIONS

| | |
|---|---|
| Appetite suppressant | Obesity |
| Thermogenesis | Weight loss |
| Weight control | |

# GARLIC *(Allium sativum)*

## PART USED: *BULB*

Garlic is nature's antibiotic. It is effective against bacteria that may be resistant to other antibiotics, and it stimulates the lymphatic system to throw off waste materials. Unlike other antibiotics, however, garlic does not destroy the body's normal flora. Instead, it has the ability to stimulate cell growth and activity, thus rejuvenating all body functions. It opens up blood vessels and reduces hypertension. Garlic is a health-building and disease-preventing herb. It is rich in potassium, zinc, vitamins A and C, and selenium, which is closely related to vitamin E in biological activity. It also contains sulphur, calcium, manganese, copper, vitamin B1, and some iron.

## PRIMARY APPLICATIONS

Asthma
Digestive disorders
High blood pressure
Cancer immunity
Ear infections
Infectious diseases

## SECONDARY APPLICATIONS

Anemia
Allergies
Cold congestion
Emphysema
Germ killer
Hypertension
Infections
Memory
Parasites
Skin problems
Toxic metal poisoning
Worms
Arthritis
Catarrh
Diabetes
Fevers
Heart disease
Hypoglycemia
Insomnia
Mucus
Regulator of glands
Toothache
Warts
Yeast infection

# GENTIAN (*Gentiana lutea*)

## PART USED: ROOT

Gentian improves circulation and stimulates the appetite, so is helpful for convalescing patients. It is also one of the best stomach tonics in the herb kingdom. It can help to improve weak muscular tone of digestive organs, and does not cause constipation. Gentian is rich is natural sugar and is useful for strengthening the pancreas, spleen, and kidneys. Gentian is high in iron. It also contains B-complex vitamins (especially inositol and niacin), vitamin F, manganese, silicon, sulphur, tin, lead, and zinc.

## PRIMARY APPLICATIONS

| | |
|---|---|
| Appetite stimulant | Hysteria |
| Jaundice | Liver bile |

## SECONDARY APPLICATIONS

| | |
|---|---|
| Amenorrhea | Anemia |
| Antidote for poison | Blood (strengthens) |
| Bruises | Constipation |
| Cramps | Debility |
| Diarrhea | Female weakness |
| Fevers | Gout |
| Heartburn | Joint inflammation |
| Nausea | Scrogula |
| Spleen disorders | Stomach problems |
| Sprains | Urinary infection |
| Vermin | Wounds (infected) |

# GINGER *(Zingiber officinale)*

*PART USED:* ROOT

Ginger is an excellent herb for the respiratory system. It is good for fighting off colds and flu, relieves headaches and other aches and pains, removes congestion, and helps to eliminate sore throats. Ginger and capsicum work together to relieve bronchial congestion and stuffy noses. Ginger is also an excellent remedy for upset stomach and indigestion. It is very effective as a cleansing agent, working through the bowels, kidneys and skin. Ginger is good for combining with other herbs because it enhances their effectiveness. It can also be added to meat dishes because it helps the intestines to detoxify the meat. Ginger contains protein, vitamins A, B-complex, C, and calcium, phosphorus, iron, sodium, potassium and magnesium.

## PRIMARY APPLICATIONS

| | |
|---|---|
| Childhood diseases | Circulation |
| Colds | Colic |
| Fevers | Flu |
| Gas Pains | Headache |
| Indigestion | Morning sickness |
| Nausea | Toothache |

## SECONDARY APPLICATIONS

| | |
|---|---|
| Bowels (spasms) | Bronchitis |
| Colitis | Coughs |
| Diarrhea | Dropsy |
| Female obstruction | Heart palpitations |
| Lung problems | Menstruation (promotes) |
| Throat, sore | Perspiration (promotes) |

# GINKGO *(Ginkgo biloba)*

## PART USED: LEAVES

Ginkgo was termed "good for the heart and lungs" in China's first great herbal book. It was introduced into Europe as early as 1730. Recent studies in Europe have found that ginkgo helps prevent strokes by preventing the formation of blood clots. Its ability to inhibit the clumping of blood platelets is beneficial because clumps and clots contribute to heart problems, strokes and artery disease. French scientists have gotten positive results when using ginkgo to promote natural blood clotting and arterial blood flow. It has also been shown to help prevent asthma attacks and organ transplant rejection. This herb strengthens arteries in the legs and relieves pain, cramping and weakness. By increasing circulation it prevents muscular degeneration.

Ginkgo is a gift for the aging individual. Ear problems are improved with ginkgo, due to improved blood flow to nerves of the inner ear. Ginkgo increases oxygen and blood flow to the brain and extremities, improves mental clarity and inhibits free radical scavengers from destroying cells. It supplies nutritional support to all areas of the body by dilating the blood vessels, allowing improved blood flow to the tissues. Ginkgo is an adaptogen herb, which helps the body deal with stressful situations.

## PRIMARY APPLICATIONS

| | |
|---|---|
| Alzheimer's disease | Attention span |
| Circulatory disorders | Dizziness |
| Memory loss | Stroke |

## SECONDARY APPLICATIONS

| | |
|---|---|
| Allergies | Alertness |
| Anxiety attacks | Arthritis |
| Asthma | Cancer |

Coughs
Equilibrium problems
Heart problems
Mental clarity
Muscular degeneration
Tinnitus
Varicose veins
Vertigo

Depression
Headaches
Lung problems
Mood swings
Raynaud's disease
Toxic shock syndrome
Vascular impotence

# GINSENG

*Korean Ginseng (Panax schin-seng)*
*Siberian Ginseng (Eleutherococcus)*
*Wild American Ginseng (panax quinquefolium)*

PART USED: ROOT

Ginseng is called "the king of herbs" in the Orient. It stimulates the entire body to overcome stress, fatigue, and weakness. It is especially good for mental fatigue because it stimulates and improves brain cells. Ginseng has a very beneficial effect on the heart and circulation. It is used to normalize blood pressure, reduce blood cholesterol and prevent arteriosclerosis.

Ginseng acts as an antidote to various types of drugs and toxic chemicals, and is said to protect the body against radiation. It works to improve vision and hearing, and help to check irritability. It is used as a preventive tonic in China and is claimed to slow down the aging process. Basically, it is considered a cure-all herb. Ginseng contains vitamins A and E. It also contains thiamine, riboflavin, B12, niacin, calcium, iron, phosphorus, sodium, silicon, potassium, manganese, magnesium, sulphur, and tin

## PRIMARY APPLICATIONS

Age spots
Depression

Blood diseases
Endurance (increases)

Hemorrhage
Physical vigor
Stress

Longevity
Sexual stimulant

## SECONDARY APPLICATIONS

Anemia
Appetite
Blood pressure
Digestive problems
Fatigue (banishes)
Inflammation
Liver diseases
Menopause
Mental vigor
Nervousness
Ulcers

Antidote for some drugs
Bleeding, internal
Childbirth (bleeding)
Euphoria (induces)
Fevers
Irritability (helps)
Lung problems
Menstruation
Nausea
Radiation protection
Vomiting

# GLUCOMANNAN

*(Amorphophallus konjak)*
PART USED: ROOT

Glucomannan, part of the same family as the yam, is a 100 percent natural source of dietary fiber—without calories. Since lack of fiber is a major cause for the high incidence of growing gastrointestinal disorders, glucomannan is a valuable herb. Besides being high in fiber, glucomannan helps reduce cholesterol, maintain regularity and promote bowel health. It helps to normalize blood sugar, to relieve stress on the pancreas and to discourage blood sugar abnormalities, such as hypoglycemia. Glucomannan absorbs toxic substances produced during digestion and elimination. It binds toxic material and eliminates them before they can be absorbed into the blood stream.

It has been found in clinical studies that glucomannan and lecithin used together are good supplements for reducing cholesterol levels. Lecithin breaks down fat and cholesterol, while glucomannan eliminates them from the body. Glucomannan expands to about 50 times its original volume when used with a large glass of water, so is a wonderful diet aid. This herb contains vitamins A, C, niacin, B1 and B2. It also contains calcium, magnesium, phosphorus, potassium, sodium, iron, zinc, selenium, manganese and silicon.

## PRIMARY APPLICATIONS

| | |
|---|---|
| Constipation | Diverticular disease |
| Hemorrhoids | Obesity |

## SECONDARY APPLICATIONS

| | |
|---|---|
| Atherosclerosis | Diabetes |
| Digestive problems | High blood pressure |
| Hypoglycemia | Pancreas (reduces stress) |

# GOLDENSEAL (Hydrastis canadensis)

## PARTS USED: RHIZOME AND ROOT

Goldenseal has been recommended as a way of boosting a sluggish glandular system and promoting hormone harmony. This herb has constituents that enter the bloodstream and help regulate liver functions. It also has a natural antibiotic ability to stop infection and kill poisons in the body.

Goldenseal is valuable for all catarrhal conditions, either in the nasal area, bronchial tubes, throat, intestines, stomach or bladder. It has the ability to heal mucous membranes anywhere in the body. It ranks high as one of the best general medicinal aids in the herbal kingdom, and can be used for ailments too numerous to mention here. When taken with other herbs, it increases their tonic properties. If a person has a low blood sugar, myrrh can be used instead of goldenseal. This herb contains vitamins A, C, B-complex, E and F, calcium, copper, potassium, phosphorus, manganese, iron, zinc and sodium. Note: Goldenseal should not be used by pregnant women.

### PRIMARY APPLICATIONS

| | |
|---|---|
| Antibiotic | Antiseptic |
| Bleeding, internal | Colon inflammation |
| Eye infections | Hemorrhaging, internal |
| Infection | Liver problems |
| Menstruation, excessive | Mouth sores |
| Vaginitis | |

### SECONDARY APPLICATIONS

| | |
|---|---|
| Cancer | Catarrh |
| Constipation, chronic | Eczema |
| Gastritis | Genital disorders |
| Gonorrhea | Herpes simplex, genital |
| Insect repellent | Morning sickness |
| Ringworm | Rhinitis |
| Skin problems | Tonsillitis |
| Ulceration, skin | Urethritis |
| Venereal disease | |

# GOTU KOLA (Hydrocotyule asiatica)

### PARTS USED: ENTIRE PLANT

Gotu kola is an herb that helps rebuild energy reserves. For this reason, it is called "food for the brain." It increases mental and physical power, combats stress and improves reflexes. Because gotu kola has an energizing effect on brain cells, it is also said to help prevent nervous breakdowns. It works to relieve high blood pressure, mental fatigue, senility, and helps the body defend itself against various toxins. Gotu kola contains vitamins A, G, K, and is high in magnesium. It probably contains vitamins E, B and minerals, but at this point no research has been done in the United States.

## PRIMARY APPLICATIONS

| | |
|---|---|
| Fatigue | High blood pressure |
| Mental fatigue | Nervous Breakdown |
| Physical fatigue | |

## SECONDARY APPLICATIONS

| | |
|---|---|
| Blood purifier | Bowel problems |
| Depression | Fevers |
| Heart (strengthens) | Infections |
| Leprosy | Longevity |
| Memory | Menopause |
| Rheumatism | Scrofula |
| Senility | Thyroid stimulant |
| Tonic | Toxins (defense) |
| Vitality | Wounds |

# GUM WEED (*Grindelia squarrosa*)

## PARTS USED: FLOWERING TOP AND LEAVES

Gum weed is mainly used as an antidote to treat poison oak and ivy, as well as other skin disorders. It has also been used to reduce the spasms, bronchial irritations and nasal congestion that accompany asthma and whooping cough. Gum weed is high in selenium. It also contains lead and traces of arsenic, tin, cadmium and zinc. Note: Individuals with weak hearts should not use gum weed.

## PRIMARY APPLICATIONS

| | |
|---|---|
| Asthma | Bronchitis |
| Bladder infection | Poison ivy and oak |
| Psoriasis | Skin disorders |

## SECONDARY APPLICATIONS

| | |
|---|---|
| Blisters, external | Burns, external |
| Dermatitis, allergic | Eczema/Impetigo |
| Emphysema | Flu |

# GYMNEMA (Gymnema sylvestre)

## PARTS USED: LEAVES AND ROOTS

Gymnema has been used for hundreds of years by Ayurvedic physicians in India to treat diabetes. Indians call this herb *gurmar,* a Hindu word meaning "sugar destroyer." Modern scientific research has confirmed that the active ingredient of the herb, gymnemic acid, blocks not only the taste of sugar, but also the absorption of sugar by the body. It is also thought that gymnema suppresses the taste of saccharin and cyclamate, two common artificial sweeteners. Another promising discovery for individuals suffering from diabetes is that gymnema has been found to increase liver and pancreatic function. This herb can also help with obesity, hypoglycemia, anemia and osteoporosis.

## PRIMARY APPLICATIONS

| | |
|---|---|
| Diabetes | Hyperactivity |
| Hypoglycemia | |

## SECONDARY APPLICATIONS

| | |
|---|---|
| Allergies | Anemia |
| Cholesterol | Digestion |
| Obesity | Weight control |

# HAWTHORN (*Crategnus oxyacantha*)

## PARTS USED: LEAVES AND BERRIES

*H*awthorn is an effective herb for relieving insomnia and nervousness. It also has strong drawing powers. In fact, poultices of crushed leaves or fruit have been used in England for centuries to treat embedded thorns, splinters, felons and whitlows. Regular use of the hawthorn fruit can strengthen heart muscles. This herb has been used in preventing arteriosclerosis and in helping such conditions as heart valve defects, an enlarged heart, angina pectoris, and difficult breathing due to ineffective heart action and lack of oxygen in the blood. Some herbalists recommend hawthorn as a preventive herb—taking it can combat diseases before actual symptoms are manifest. Hawthorn is high in vitamins C and B-complex. It contains sodium, silicon, phosphorus, and smaller amounts of iron, zinc, sulphur, nickel, tin, aluminum and veryllium.

## PRIMARY APPLICATIONS

| | |
|---|---|
| Antiseptic | Arteriosclerosis (prevents) |
| Cardiac symptoms | Enlarged heart |
| Hardening of the arteries | Heart palpitation |
| High blood pressure | Hypoglycemia |

## SECONDARY APPLICATIONS

| | |
|---|---|
| Angina | Arthritis |
| Congestive heart failure | Dropsy |
| Insomnia | Kidney trouble |
| Low blood pressure | Miscarriage |
| Rheumatism, inflammatory | Throat, sore |

# HOPS (*Humulus lupulus*)

## PART USED: FLOWER

Hops is recognized for its remarkable sedative powers. It is known as one of the best nervines in the herb kingdom for overcoming insomnia. Its main uses are to alleviate nervous tension and promote restful sleep. It also stimulates the glands and muscles of the stomach while at the same time calming the hyperexcitable gastric nerves. It has a relaxing influence upon the liver and gall ducts and works as a laxative. Hops is rich in the B-complex vitamin. It also contains magnesium, zinc, copper, traces of iodine, manganese, iron, sodium, lead, fluorine, and chlorine.

## PRIMARY APPLICATIONS

Appetite stimulant
Delirium
Headaches
Insomnia
Pain

Bronchitis
Digestion
Hyperactivity
Nervousness
Sexual desires, excessive

## SECONDARY APPLICATIONS

Blood cleanser
Cramps, abdominal
Earache
Fevers, high
Hysteria
Jaundice
Neuralgia
Toothache
Water retention

Bruises
Dizziness
Female problems
Gallstones
Itching
Kidney stones
Skin irritations
Venereal disease
Whooping cough

# HOREHOUND *(Marrubium vulgare)*

PARTS USED: ENTIRE PLANT

Horehound is well known as a cure for children's coughs, croup and colds. This herb's expectorant properties assist in loosening tough phlegm from the chest. Warm infusions will relieve congestion and hyperemic conditions of the lungs by promoting an outward flow of blood. In large doses, horehound acts as a laxative. Applying the dried herb topically has been recommended for use with herpes simplex, eruptions, eczema and shingles. Horehound contains vitamins A, E, C, F and B-complex, iron, potassium, and sulphur.

## PRIMARY APPLICATIONS

| | |
|---|---|
| Asthma | Colds/Coughs |
| Lungs | Phlegm |
| Respiratory organs | Croup |

## SECONDARY APPLICATIONS

| | |
|---|---|
| Bronchitis | Earaches |
| Eczema, external | Fevers |
| Glands (stimulates) | Infectious diseases |
| Jaundice | Laxative, mild |
| Menstruation (produces) | Shingles, external |
| Stomach tonic | Sweating (promotes) |

# HORSERADISH *(Cochlearia armoracia)*

PART USED: ROOT

Horseradish has an antibiotic action which is recommended for respiratory and urinary infections. It has been used internally to clear nasal passages and cleanse various body systems. It has also been used to stimulate digestion, metabolism and kidney function. Horseradish is rich in vitamins C and B1, sulphur, and potassium. It also contains vitamins A, P and B-complex, iron, calcium, phosphorus and sodium.

## PRIMARY APPLICATIONS

Appetite stimulant
Circulation
Dropsy
Tumors, skin and internal

Catarrh
Cough
Sinus problems
Worms (expel)

## SECONDARY APPLICATIONS

Arthritis, external
Bronchitis
Gout
Kidney
Neuralgia, external
Rheumatism
Water retention

Asthma
Congestion
Jaundice
Mucous membrane
Palsy
Skin
Wounds, septic

# HORSETAIL (*Equisetum arvense*)

## PARTS USED: ENTIRE PLANT

Horsetail (or shavegrass) is used in urinary tract disorders, especially lower tract infections. The most important ingredient in the herb is silicic acid, which helps circulation. Horsetail aids in coagulation so a decoction applied externally will help staunch and heal bleeding wounds. Research has shown that fractured bones will heal much faster when horsetail is taken. This herb is rich in silicon and selenium. It also contains vitamin E, pantothenic acid, PABA, copper, manganese, sodium, cobalt, iron, and iodine.

## PRIMARY APPLICATIONS

| | |
|---|---|
| Bladder problems | Bleeding, internal |
| Circulation problems | Glandular disorders |
| Nails, brittle | Nosebleeds |
| Urinary ulcers | Urination, suppressed |

## SECONDARY APPLICATIONS

| | |
|---|---|
| Dropsy | Fever |
| Kidney problems | Liver, overactive |
| Menstruation, excess | Nervous tension |
| Skin rashes | Tuberculosis, pulmonary |

# HO-SHOU-WU *(Polygonum multiflorum)*

### PART USED: ROOT

Ho-shou-wu is said to improve health, stamina, and resistance to diseases. It is a member of the smartweed family. (Knotweed, bistort and buckwheat are memebers of the same family.) This herb has a toning effect on the liver and kidneys. It helps the nervous system and can be used as a tonic for the endocrine glands. Ho-shou-wu has properties comparable with those of ginseng. It is useful for premature graying of hair, backache, aches and pains of the knee joint, neurasthenia, and traumatic bruises.

## PRIMARY APPLICATIONS

| | |
|---|---|
| Fertility | Hair, premature graying |
| Muscles | Nerves |

## SECONDARY APPLICATIONS

| | |
|---|---|
| Anemia | Backache |
| Blood, strengthens | Bones |
| Bruises | Cancer |

Constipation
Diarrhea
Hypoglycemia
Kidneys
Liver weakness
Scrofula
Tumors

Diabetes
Fever
Insomnia
Knee (pains and ligaments)
Menstrual problems
Spleen weakness
Vertigo

# HYDRANGEA (*Hydrangea arborescens*)

## PARTS USED: LEAVES AND ROOT

*H*ydrangea is a remarkable herb. Its curative properties are second to no other plant. It contains alkaloids that act like cortisone and it has the same cleansing power of chaparral. Hydrangea is useful for preventing the formation of gravel deposits. It is also known to relieve pain when already formed gravel formations pass from the kidneys to the bladder. Hydrangea contains calcium, potassium, sodium, sulphur, phosphorus, iron, and magnesium.

## PRIMARY APPLICATIONS

Arthritis
Gallstones
Gout
Rheumatism

Bladder infections
Gonorrhea
Kidney stones
Urinary problems

## SECONDARY APPLICATIONS

Arteriosclerosis
Calculi
Pain

Backaches
Kidney problems
Renal irritations

# HYSSOP *(Hyssopus officinalis)*

*PART USED: LEAVES*

Hyssop is used for lung ailments and fevers. Research has found that the mold which produces penicillin grows on hyssop leaves and adds to the herb's healing powers. Hyssop also contains essential hormone oils which help build resistance to infectious diseases. The leaves can be placed directly on wounds to stop infections and aid in healing. This herb has also been used for poor digestion, breast and lung problems, coughs, colds and nose and throat infections. Hyssop is usually mixed with other herbs for best results.

## PRIMARY APPLICATIONS

| | |
|---|---|
| Catarrh, chronic | Congestion |
| Coughs, irritable | Lung ailments |
| Phlegm, hard | Throat, sore |

## SECONDARY APPLICATIONS

| | |
|---|---|
| Asthma | Blood pressure |
| Bronchitis | Bruises |
| Colds | Cuts |
| Rheumatism | Ear ailments |
| Epilepsy | Fevers |
| Jaundice | Kidney/Liver problems |

# ICELAND MOSS *(Cetraria islandica)*

*PARTS USED: ENTIRE PLANT*

Iceland moss is really not a moss, but a lichen. It has been known for centuries as a cure for all kinds of chest ailments. It is used to nourish sickly children, invalids and aged persons. Iceland moss has the same properties as Irish moss, so the vitamin and mineral content are probably about the same. This herb is high in iodine, calcium, potassium and phosphorus.

### PRIMARY APPLICATIONS

Anemia

Catarrh

Coughs

Lung problems

Bronchitis

Congestion

Digestive troubles

### SECONDARY APPLICATIONS

Diarrhea

Fevers

Hoarseness

Tuberculosis

Dysentery

Gastritis

Lactation

# IRISH MOSS (*Chondrus crispus*)

### PARTS USED: ENTIRE PLANT

Irish moss is a very useful herb for those recovering from illness because of its high nutrient content. It also has a high mucilage content which helps sooth inflamed tissues and reduce lung and kidney problems. Irish moss has been used externally to soften skin and prevent wrinkles. It purifies and strengthens the cellular structure and vital fluids of the system. This herb contains small and usable quantities of iodine, which contributes to the health of the body's glandular system. Healthy glands are beneficial for all functions of the body. Irish moss contains vitamins A, D, E, F and K. It is high in iodine, calcium and sodium and has some phosphorus, potassium and sulphur. It is worth noting that this herb contains fifteen of the eighteen elements which compose the human body.

## PRIMARY APPLICATIONS

| | |
|---|---|
| Bronchitis | Thyroid |
| Goiter | Lung problems |

## SECONDARY APPLICATIONS

| | |
|---|---|
| Bladder problems | Cancer |
| Halitosis | Intestinal problems |
| Joints, swollen | Tuberculosis |
| Tumors | Ulcers, peptic |
| Varicose veins | |

# JOJOBA (*Simmondsia chinensis*)

## PART USED: OIL

Jojoba oil, made from the seeds of the plant, has traditionally been used by Native Americans to promote hair growth and relieve skin problems. Scientists have found that deposits of sebum tend to collect and solidify around hair follicles causing dandruff, hair loss and scalp disorders. Jojoba oil removes the embedded sebum and makes the scalp less acidic. Jojoba contains vitamins E and B-complex, silicon, chromium, copper, zinc, and is rich in iodine.

## PRIMARY APPLICATIONS

| | |
|---|---|
| Chapped skin | Dandruff |
| Hair loss | Psoriasis |
| Scalp, dry | Skin, dry |

## SECONDARY APPLICATIONS

| | |
|---|---|
| Abrasions | Acne (vulgaris) |
| Athletes foot | Cuts |
| Eczema | Mouth sores |
| Pimples | Seborrhea |
| Warts | Wrinkles |

# JUNIPER *(Juniperis species)*

## PART USED: BERRIES

Juniper is high in natural insulin and has the ability to restore the pancreas when there has been no permanent damage. It is excellent for infections and disease prevention. It is also good for disorders that cause uric acid to be retained in the body. This herb is high in vitamin C and cobalt. It contains sulphur, copper, and a trace of tin and aluminum.

## PRIMARY APPLICATIONS

Bleeding
Infections
Pancreas
Urinary disorders

Colds
Kidney infections
Uric acid, build up
Water retention

## SECONDARY APPLICATIONS

Ague
Colic
Convulsions
Diabetes
Gonorrhea
Insect bites, poisonous
Menstruation (regulates)

Bladder problems
Coughs
Cramps
Gas
Gums, bleeding
Leucorrhea
Snakebites

# KAVA KAVA *(Piper methysticum)*

## PART USED: ROOT

Kava kava is used by Polynesians in their ceremonial drinks because it brings a sense of well-being, calms nervous anxiety, and helps to fight fatigue. It is considered an important herb for pain relief. Kava kava is recommended as a muscle relaxant because research done with animals has found the herb to contain anticonvulsant and muscle relaxing properties. Kava kava is used as an analgesic sedative for rheumatism and insomnia. It has antiseptic properties to help with bladder infections and may be directly applied to wounds.

## PRIMARY APPLICATIONS

Insomnia                    Nervousness

## SECONDARY APPLICATIONS

Anxiety                     Asthma
Bronchitis                  Fatigue
Pain                        Rheumatism
Urinary Infections          Vaginitis
Venereal Disease

# KELP *(Fucus versiculosus)*

## PARTS USED: ENTIRE PLANT

Kelp is a good promoter of glandular health. It controls the thyroid and regulates/stimulates the metabolism. Kelp has the reputation of speeding up the burning of excess calories and is helpful in the nourishment of the body. It contains all of the minerals considered vital to health. It even contains a small amount of lecithin. Kelp has a beneficial effect on many disorders of the body. It works to sustain the nervous system and helps the brain to function normally. It is essential during pregnancy.

Kelp contains nearly thirty minerals. It is rich in iodine, calcium, sulphur and silicon. It also contains phosphorus, iron, sodium, potassium, magnesium, chlorine, copper, zinc and manganese. It has a small amount of barium, boron, chromium, lithium, nickel, silver, titanium, vanadium, aluminum, strontium, bismuth, chlorine, cobalt, gallium, tin and zirconium. Kelp is rich in B-complex vitamins and contains vitamin A, C, E, G, the antisterility vitamin S, and the antihemorrhage vitamin K.

## PRIMARY APPLICATIONS

Adrenal glands
Colitis
Eczema
Goiter
Pituitary gland

Arteries (cleans)
Complexion
Fingernails
Obesity
Thyroid gland

## SECONDARY APPLICATIONS

Asthma
Diabetes
Gallbladder
Headaches
Kidneys
Nervous disorder
Pancreas
Skin
Vitality, low
Wrinkles

Constipation
Digestion, poor
Gas
High blood pressure
Morning sickness
Neuritis
Prostate (tones)
Uterus, weak
Water retention

# LADY'S SLIPPER *(Cypripedium pubescens)*

## PART USED: ROOT

Lady's slipper acts as a tonic for an exhausted nervous system. It has a calming effect on the body and mind. It is said to be one of the best and safest nervines in the plant kingdom. This means it can be used for sickly and nervous children. Its action is slow, yet effective. Lady's slipper acts primarily on the medulla, helping to regulate breathing, sweating, saliva and heart functions. It is an excellent pain reliever. This herb contains the B-complex vitamins.

PRIMARY APPLICATIONS

| | |
|---|---|
| Chorea | Hysteria |
| Insomnia | Nervousness |
| Restlessness | |

SECONDARY APPLICATIONS

| | |
|---|---|
| Abdominal pain | After pains |
| Colic | Cramps |
| Cystic fibrosis | Epilepsy |
| Headaches, nervous | Muscle spasms |
| Neuralgia | Pain |
| Tremors | Typhoid fever |

# LEMON GRASS (Cymbopogon citratus)

PART USED: LEAVES

*L*emon grass has an astringent or tightening effect on tissues of the body. This helps to stop or slow discharge from mucous membranes, which makes the herb useful for infants and children. It is a mild herb, which also makes it an excellent remedy for people under stress and for women suffering from cramps, headaches and dizziness. Lemon grass tea is used to relieve colds, flu and fevers. The herb is very high in vitamins A and C.

PRIMARY APPLICATIONS

| | |
|---|---|
| Colds | Digestion |
| Fevers | |

SECONDARY APPLICATIONS

| | |
|---|---|
| Bladder | Boils (warm poultice) |
| Colic | Gas |
| Headaches | High blood pressure |
| Insect bites | Kidneys |

Liver

Nausea

Spleen

Menstruation, suppressed

Nervousness

Vomiting

# LICORICE *(Glycyrrhiza glabra)*

## PART USED: ROOT

*L*icorice is a source of the female hormone, estrogen. This makes it a very important herb for female complaints. Another important property of licorice is that it works to stimulate the adrenal glands. Such stimulation helps counteract stress and supplies energy to the body, making licorice an important herb for those recovering from illness. Licorice also contains glycosides which can chemically purge excess fluid from the lungs, throat and body. It has long been recognized as a remedy for coughs and other chest complaints. This herb also works as a laxative, helps to reduce inflammation of the intestinal tract, and helps to relieve ulcer conditions. Licorice contains vitamins E and B-complex, phosphorus, biotin, niacin, and pantothenic acid. It also has lecithin, manganese, iodine, chromium, and zinc.

## PRIMARY APPLICATIONS

Addison's disease

Colds

Drug withdrawal

Female complaints

Hypoglycemia

Phlegm (expels)

Tonic

Blood cleanser

Cough

Energy

Hoarseness

Lung problems

Throat (sore)

## SECONDARY APPLICATIONS

Adrenal exhaustion

Arteriosclerosis

Age spots

Arthritis

Bronchial congestion
Constipation
Emphysema
Fevers
Heart (strengthens)
Liver

Circulation
Cushing's disease
Endurance
Flu
Impotency
Ulcers

# LILY-OF-THE-VALLEY

*(Convallaria majalis)*
PARTS USED: FLOWER, LEAF, AND RHIZOME

Lily-of-the-valley has been recommended by Dr. Edward Shook as a valuable cardiac tonic. He suggests it for slowing the action of the heart and increasing the force of heart contractions. Lily-of-the-valley contains twenty cardiac glycosides and works on heart disorders much the same as digitalis, but without the side effects. It can also help reduce water retention, which often accompanies heart problems, and works to strengthen the heart and the arteries. Lily-of-the-valley has also been used to treat brain weakness and memory problems. In Europe it is used extensively for apoplexy, epilepsy, heart ailments, palsy, and vertigo.

Lily-of-the-valley contains potassium, which is effective in dissolving fibrous and catarrhal matter. Its calcium content is essential for the heart. It contains iron, which strengthens the blood and helps slow the growth of varicose ulcers and veins, tumors, cancers, ulcerated gums and gangrene. The herb also contains rutin which helps strengthen the vascular system, especially the capillaries.

## PRIMARY APPLICATIONS

Arrhythmia
Heart disorders
Epilepsy

Edema
Water retention

# LOBELIA *(Lobelia inflata)*

*PARTS USED: ENTIRE PLANT*

*L*obelia is a valuable herb. It is the most powerful relaxant in the herb kingdom, and modern use has shown that it has no harmful effects. Its healing powers include the ability to remove congestion within the body, especially from the blood vessels. It is also good for bronchial spasms. Lobelia can be used externally in a poultice with slippery elm and a little soap to bring abscesses or boils to a head. Lobelia contains sulphur, iron, cobalt, selenium, sodium, copper, and lead.

## PRIMARY APPLICATIONS

Arthritis (tincture)
Bronchitis
Colds
Convulsions
Croup (tincture)
Ear infections
Fevers
Lock jaw (tincture)
Miscarriage
Pain
Whooping cough

Asthma
Catarrh
Congestion
Cough
Earache (tincture)
Epilepsy
Food Poisoning
Lung problems
Nervousness
Pneumonia
Worms

## SECONDARY APPLICATIONS

Allergies
Childhood diseases
Colic
Eczema
Headache
Hepatitis
Palsy
Poison ivy and oak

Blood poisoning
Circulation
Constipation
Female problems
Heart
Hydrophobia
Pleurisy
Rheumatism

Rabies                    Ringworm (tincture)
Scarlet fever             Shock
Spasms                    Syphilis
Teeth                     Tetanus
Tonsillitis               Toothaches
Vomiting (small doses)    Wounds

# MANDRAKE (*Podophylluim peltatum*)

PART USED: ROOT

Mandrake (the American variety) is a very strong glandular stimulant. It is used for chronic liver diseases, skin problems, bile flow, digestion, and the elimination of obstructions. Mandrake is often combined with supporting herbs to regulate liver and bowels, for uterine disorders and intermittent fevers. It is being studied as a natural plant cure for cancer. It is a powerful herb and should be used with caution. It should not be used during pregnancy.

## PRIMARY APPLICATIONS

Bowels, lower             Cancer
Constipation              Fevers
Indigestion               Liver problems
Worms

## SECONDARY APPLICATIONS

Asthma                    Diarrhea
Gallstones                Hayfever
Headaches                 Jaundice
Lead poisoning            Nervousness
Pain, chronic             Rheumatism
Scrofula                  Skin problems
Syphilis                  Typhoid fever
Vomiting                  Warts

# MARIGOLD *(Calendula officinalis)*

*PARTS USED: ENTIRE PLANT*

**M**arigold is very useful as a first aid remedy. Marigold tea is used to relieve acute ailments, especially fevers. A tincture of marigold is good for bruises, sprains, muscle spasms, and ulcers. A marigold poultice is useful for bleeding hemorrhoids. Marigold has also been used as a snuff to discharge mucus from the nose. It is said by some herbalists to be excellent for the heart and for circulation. This herb is high in phosphorus and contains vitamins A and C.

## PRIMARY APPLICATIONS

| | |
|---|---|
| Bruises, external | Cuts, external |
| Eye infections | Skin diseases |

## SECONDARY APPLICATIONS

| | |
|---|---|
| Amenorrhea | Anemia |
| Blood cleansers | Bronchitis |
| Cancer | Colitis |
| Cramps | Diarrhea |
| Ear infections | Fevers |
| Hemorrhoids | Hepatitis |
| Jaundice | Ulcers |
| Varicose veins | Wounds |

# MARJORAM *(Origanum vulgare)*

*PARTS USED: ENTIRE PLANT*

**M**arjoram has stimulant and carminative properties. These make the herb useful for conditions like asthma, coughs and various spasmodic afflictions. Marjoram helps to strengthen the stomach and intestines and is also used as an antidote for narcotic poisons, convulsions and dropsy. It contains vitamins A and C, niacin, some thiamine, riboflavin, and vitamin B12. It has also has calcium, potassium, magnesium, phosphorus, some iron, sodium, zinc, and silicon.

## PRIMARY APPLICATIONS

| | |
|---|---|
| Colic | Coughs, violent |
| Cramps, abdominal | Headaches, nervous |
| Indigestion | Respiratory problems |

## SECONDARY APPLICATIONS

| | |
|---|---|
| Asthma | Bedwetting |
| Convulsions | Diarrhea |
| Dropsy | Fevers |
| Gas | Gastritis |
| Measles (regulate) | Narcotic poisoning |
| Nightmares | Nausea |
| Neuralgia | Seasickness |
| Toothaches (oil) | Water retention |

# MARSHMALLOW (Althaea officinalis)

PART USED: ROOT

Marshmallow contains mucilage which helps expectorate difficult phlegm and relax the bronchial tubes. The soothing and healing properties of marshmallow mucilage make the herb valuable for many lung ailments, especially asthma. Marshmallow is also a powerful anti-inflammatory and anti-irritant which makes it good for joints and gastrointestinal disorders. Marshmallow heals the irritations associated with diarrhea and dysentery. Used externally as a poultice with cayenne, it can be used to treat blood poisoning, gangrene, burns, bruises, and wounds. Marshmallow contains 286,000 units of vitamin A per pound. It is also rich in calcium and zinc and has iron, sodium, iodine, B-complex, and pantothenic acid.

## PRIMARY APPLICATIONS

| | |
|---|---|
| Asthma | Bleeding, urinary |
| Boils | Bronchial infections |
| Emphysema | Kidneys |
| Lung congestion | Wounds, infected |

## SECONDARY APPLICATIONS

| | |
|---|---|
| Breast problems | Burns (acid or fire) |
| Catarrh | Constipation |
| Cough, dry | Diabetes |
| Diarrhea | Dysentery |
| Eyes, sore | Glands |
| Gravel | Intestines |
| Lactation | Liver problems |
| Mucous membranes | Skin |
| Stomach problems | Throat, sore |
| Urinary infections | |

# MILK THISTLE (*Silybum marianum*)

## PART USED: SEEDS

Milk thistle plays a major role in protecting, rejuvenating and restoring liver function. It was used centuries ago by the Romans for restoring impaired liver function and is currently being used in Europe for the same reason. Milk thistle is an excellent treatment for liver disease because it can block damage to and regenerate liver cells. In this way, it affects the whole body because the function of the liver is to protect the immune system. This herb is also an antioxidant which protects against free-radical scavengers. It works to prevent plaque buildup and the hardening of arteries. Milk thistle is rich in bioflavonoids and stimulates protein synthesis.

## PRIMARY APPLICATIONS

| | |
|---|---|
| Gallbladder problems | Liver damage |
| Spleen | Stomach |

## SECONDARY APPLICATIONS

| | |
|---|---|
| Alcoholism | Appetite stimulant |
| Boils | Chemotherapy (protects ) |
| Cirrhosis | Depression |
| Fatty Deposits | Gas |
| Heartburn | Hepatitis |
| Indigestion | Radiation |

# MISTLETOE *(Phorandendron flavescens)*

## PARTS USED: ENTIRE PLANT

Mistletoe is one of nature's best tranquilizers and is not habit forming. It is useful for any condition involving a weakness or disorder of the nervous system. It will quiet and soothe the nerves and reduce cerebral activity, so is a good remedy for migraine headaches. Mistletoe also works on the circulatory system to constrict blood vessels and stimulate the the heart beat. Some modern European physicians believe that treating the spleen with mistletoe may be beneficial in cases of epilepsy. Mistletoe contains vitamin B12, calcium, sodium, magnesium, potassium, iron, cobalt, iodine, copper, and cadmium.

## PRIMARY APPLICATIONS

| | |
|---|---|
| Chorea | Circulation (stimulates) |
| Convulsions | Epilepsy |

Hemorrhages, internal
Menstruation
Spleen

High blood pressure
Nervousness

## SECONDARY APPLICATIONS

Arteriosclerosis
Asthma
Blood cleanser
Delirium
Heart problems
Hypoglycemia
Mental disturbance
Neuralgia
Tonic

Arthritis
Bed wetting
Cholera
Gallbladder
Hypertension
Hysteria
Migraine headaches
Rheumatism
Tumors

# MULLEIN *(Verbascum thapsus)*

## PART USED: FLOWERS AND LEAVES

Mullein has narcotic properties without being habit forming or poisonous. It is an excellent pain killer and helps induce sleep. It also has a calming effect on all inflamed and irritated nerves. This is why it works so well in controlling coughs, cramps and spasms. It has the ability to loosen mucus and move it out of the body so is valuable for all lung problems. Fresh mullein flowers can be crushed and topically applied as a remedy for warts. Mullein tea has been used for dropsy, sinusitis, and swollen joints. The hot tea also helps with mumps, tumors, sore throats, and tonsillitis. Mullein is high in iron, magnesium, potassium and sulphur. It contains vitamins A, D, and B-complex.

## PRIMARY APPLICATIONS

Asthma
Bronchitis

Bleeding (bowel and lungs)
Coughs

Croup
Earaches (oil)
Lymphatic system
Pain (relieves)
Sinus congestion

Diarrhea
Insomnia
Nervousness
Pleurisy
Tuberculosis

## SECONDARY APPLICATIONS

Bowel complaints
Colds
Diaper rash
Female problems
Glands, cleans
Hemorrhage
Hoarseness
Pneumonia
Venereal diseases

Bruises
Cramps
Dropsy
Gas
Hay fever
Hemorrhoids
Lung problems
Sores
Wounds

# MUSTARD (Sinapis alba)

### PART USED: SEEDS

Mustard is a strong, stimulating herb. It promotes appetite and stimulates the gastrate mucous membrane to help in digestion. An infusion of mustard seed stimulates urine and helps in delayed menstruation. It is also a valuable emetic for narcotic poisoning because it empties the stomach without depression of the system. Mustard is often used externally as a plaster or poultice for sore, stiff muscles. Mustard helps to loosen the muscles up and carry away toxins causing them to tighten. Mustard is an excellent source of calcium, phosphorus and potassium. It contains vitamins A, B1, B2, B12 and C. It also contains sulphur, iron, cobalt and traces of manganese and iodine.

## PRIMARY APPLICATIONS

Indigestion
Lungs

Liver

## SECONDARY APPLICATIONS

Appetite stimulant
Bad breath
Bronchitis
Feet (sore)
Gas
Pleurisy
Sore throat
Pneumonia

Arthritis
Blood purifier
Emphysema
Fever
Hiccups
Snake bites
Kidneys
Sprains

# MYRRH *(Balsamodendron myrrha)*

## PART USED: RESIN

Myrrh is a powerful antiseptic. Like echinacea, it is a valuable cleansing and healing agent. Myrrh works on stomach and colon problems by helping sooth inflammation and speeding the healing process. Myrrh gives vitality and strength to the digestive system and helps in waste elimination. The herb's essential oils, when used as a tincture mixed with water, are excellent as a gargle for sore throat. Myrrh has also been used with goldenseal to make a healing antiseptic salve.

## PRIMARY APPLICATIONS

Bad breath
Catarrh, chronic
Hemorrhoids
Mouth sores
Stomach (cleans)

Bronchitis
Colon (cleans)
Lung diseases
Skin sores
Throat, sore

## SECONDARY APPLICATIONS

| | |
|---|---|
| Abrasions | Asthma |
| Bed sores | Coughs |
| Cuts | Diarrhea, chronic |
| Eczema | Gas |
| Gums | Herpes |
| Indigestion | Menstrual problems |
| Nipples, sore | Pimples |
| Sinus problems | Tuberculosis |
| Ulcers | Wounds |

# NETTLE (Urtica dioica)

### PART USED: LEAVES AND ROOT

Nettle has long been recognized as one of the most useful of all plants. This knowledge has come from centuries of experience. The plant contains alkaloids that neutralize uric acid. It is now understood that decreasing uric acid helps reduce symptoms of rheumatism. Nettle is also rich in iron which is vital to good circulation and helps reduce high blood pressure. Tannin found in the nettle root has been used as part of an astringent enema to shrink hemorrhoids and reduce excess menstrual flow. Nettle is so rich in chlorophyll that the English used it to make the green dye used in World War II camouflage paint. It is also rich in iron, silicon, and potassium, and vitamins A and C. It contains protein, vitamins E, D, F and P, calcium, sulphur, sodium, copper, manganese, chromium and zinc.

## PRIMARY APPLICATIONS

| | |
|---|---|
| Bleeding, internal | Bleeding, external |
| Blood purifier | Bronchitis |
| Diarrhea | High blood pressure |
| Rheumatism | |

## SECONDARY APPLICATIONS

| | |
|---|---|
| Anemia | Asthma |
| Circulation, poor | Eczema |
| Hemorrhoids | Hives |
| Kidneys, inflamed | Menstruation, excess |
| Mouth sores | Nosebleeds |
| Skin ailments | Vaginitis |

# OATSTRAW (Avena sativa)

## PART USED: STEMS

Oatstraw is a powerful stimulant and is rich in body-building materials. In homeopathy, a tincture made from the fresh flowering plant is used for arthritis, rheumatism, paralysis, liver infections and skin diseases. Hot oatstraw compresses relieve pain from kidney stone attacks. Oatstraw has many elements that have antiseptic properties and, when eaten frequently, is said to be a natural preventative for contagious disease. Oatstraw is high in silicon and rich in calcium. It contains phosphorus and vitamins A, B1, B2 and E.

## PRIMARY APPLICATIONS

| | |
|---|---|
| Indigestion | Nerves |
| Insomnia | Heart (strengthens) |

## SECONDARY APPLICATIONS

| | |
|---|---|
| Arthritis | Bladder |
| Boils | Bones, brittle |
| Bursitis | Constipation |
| Gout | Kidneys |
| Liver | Lungs |
| Pancreas | Paralysis |
| Rheumatism | Wounds |

# OREGON GRAPE *(Berberis aquifolium)*

*PARTS USED: RHIZOME AND ROOT*

Oregon grape is well known for treatment of skin diseases caused by toxins in the blood. This is because it stimulates the action of the liver and is one of the best blood cleansers. It also mildly stimulates thyroid functions. Oregon grape aids in the assimilation of nutrients, and is a tonic for all glands. This herb contains minerals such as manganese, silicon, sodium, copper and zinc. It can be substituted for goldenseal.

## PRIMARY APPLICATIONS

| | |
|---|---|
| Acne | Staph infections |
| Blood conditions | Digestion (promotes) |
| Eczema | Jaundice |
| Liver | Psoriasis |

## SECONDARY APPLICATIONS

| | |
|---|---|
| Arthritis, rheumatoid | Bowels |
| Bronchitis | Constipation, chronic |
| Hepatitis | Herpes |
| Kidneys | Leucorrhea |
| Lymph glands | Rheumatism |
| Strength (increases) | Syphilis |
| Uterine diseases | Vaginitis (douche) |

# PAPAYA *(Carica papaya)*

*PART USED: FRUIT, JUICE AND SEEDS*

Papaya contains papain, an enzyme that breaks down protein to a digestible state. It is good to eat this fruit after meals to help digest food. Papaya is also valued as a blood clotting agent and ulcerated skin and open wounds have been treated by wrapping them in fresh papaya leaves. Papaya seeds are given with honey for expelling worms and reducing enlargement of the liver and spleen. A paste made of the seeds can be applied to the skin to heal diseases like ringworm. Papaya juice has been used to dissolve corns, warts and pimples. Papaya contains vitamins B, D, E, G, K and C. It also contains calcium, iron, phosphorus and potassium. It is rich in sodium, magnesium, and vitamin A.

## PRIMARY APPLICATIONS

| | |
|---|---|
| Colon | Digestion |
| Gas | Insect bites |
| Intestinal tract | |

## SECONDARY APPLICATIONS

| | |
|---|---|
| Allergies | Blood clotting |
| Burns | Constipation |
| Diarrhea, chronic | Freckles (juice) |
| Hemorrhage | Sores |
| Stomach problems | Wounds |

# PARSLEY *(Petroselinum staivum)*

## PART USED: LEAVES

*P*arsley should be used as a preventive herb. It is so nutritious that it increases resistance to infections and disease. The roots and leaves are very good for all liver and spleen problems caused by jaundice and venereal diseases. Parsley is said to contain a substance in which cancerous cells cannot multiply. This possibility is being researched now. It is also known that parsley increases iron content in the blood. Parsley is high in vitamins A, B and C, potassium, iron, and chlorophyll. It contains some sodium, copper, thiamine and riboflavin, silicon, sulphur, calcium and cobalt. Note: Parsley should not be used during pregnancy, as it could bring on labor pains, and it will dry up mother's milk after birth.

## PRIMARY APPLICATIONS

| | |
|---|---|
| Bladder infections | Blood builder |
| Blood cleanser | Gallstones |
| Jaundice | Kidney inflammation |
| Urine retention | |

## SECONDARY APPLICATIONS

| | |
|---|---|
| Allergies | Arthritis |
| Asthma | Blood pressure (low) |
| Breath (bad) | Cancer |
| Coughs | Digestion (aids) |
| Conjunctivitis | Gonorrhea |
| Gout | Hay fever |
| Liver | Lumbago |
| Menstruation (promotes) | Pituitary |
| Prostate | Rheumatism |
| Sciatica | Thyroid |
| Tumors | Varicose veins |
| Venereal diseases | |

# PASSIONFLOWER (*Passiflora incarnata*)

*PARTS USED: ENTIRE PLANT*

Passionflower is used in Italy to treat hyperactive children. In the Yucatan it is used for insomnia, hysteria and convulsions in children. It works well for such conditions because it is quieting and soothing to the nervous system. It is good for unrest, agitation and exhaustion. This makes passionflower helpful for those who want to wean themselves from synthetic sleeping pills and tranquilizers. An added bonus is that this herb does not cause depression nor disorientation. It is also thought that passionflower kills a form of bacteria which causes eye irritations; therefore, it is good for inflamed eyes and dimness of vision.

## PRIMARY APPLICATIONS

|  |  |
|---|---|
| Eye infection | Fevers |
| Insomnia | Menopause |

## SECONDARY APPLICATIONS

|  |  |
|---|---|
| Asthma, spasmodic | Convulsions |
| Diarrhea | Dysentery |
| Epilepsy | Eye strain |
| Headaches | High blood pressure |
| Hysteria | Menstruation, painful |
| Muscle spasms | Nervous breakdown |
| Pain | Vision (dimness) |

# PAU D'ARCO (*Tabebuia avellanedae*)

## PART USED: INNER BARK

Pau d'arco, also known as taheebo, is an herb grown in South America. It is a powerful antibiotic with virus-killing properties. Its compounds seem to attack the very cause of disease. It is said that one of this herb's main actions is to put the body into a defensive posture, giving the energy needed to resist disease. Pau d'arco has been used on cancer patients in some hospitals in South America with great success. It contains a high amount of iron which aids in the proper assimilation of nutrients and the elimination of wastes.

## PRIMARY APPLICATIONS

|  |  |
|---|---|
| Blood purifier | Cancer, all types |
| Pain (relieves) | Skin cancer |

## SECONDARY APPLICATIONS

| | |
|---|---|
| Anemia | Arteriosclerosis |
| Asthma | Bronchitis |
| Colitis | Cystitis |
| Diabetes | Eczema |
| Eyelids (paralysis) | Fistulas |
| Gastritis | Gonorrhea |
| Hemorrhages | Hernias |
| Hodgkin's disease | Infections |
| Leukemia | Liver ailments |
| Lupus | Nephritis |
| Osteomyelitis | Parkinson's disease |
| Polyps | Prostatitis |
| Psoriasis | Rheumatism |
| Spleen infections | Syphilis |
| Ulcers | Varicose ulcers |

# PEACH (Prunus persica)

## PARTS USED: BARK AND LEAVES

Peach contains curative powers. The powdered, dried leaves have been used to heal sores and wounds. Peach contains strengthening powers for the nervous system and has mild sedative properties. It is useful for chronic bronchitis and chest complaints because of its expectorant properties. It also stimulates urine flow.

## PRIMARY APPLICATIONS

| | |
|---|---|
| Bladder | Bronchitis, chronic |
| Congestion, chest | Nausea |
| Water retention | |

## SECONDARY APPLICATIONS

| | |
|---|---|
| Constipation | Insomnia |
| Jaundice | Morning sickness |

Mucus
Sores
Uterine problems

Nervousness
Stomach problems
Whooping cough

# PENNYROYAL  *(Hedeoma Pulegioides)*

*PARTS USED: ENTIRE PLANT*

Pennyroyal contains a volatile oil which works in the stomach to remove gas. It can be taken as a tea or used as a hot footbath. If taken a few days before menstruation is due, it can help increase a suppressed flow. Pennyroyal tea is also useful for colds. This herb has a strong minty smell and is used externally to repel insects such as fleas, flies and mosquitoes. Pennyroyal contains minerals such as lead and sodium.

## PRIMARY APPLICATIONS

Bronchitis
Colds
Cramps
Fevers
Lung infections

Childbirth
Colic
Female problems
Gas
Menstruation (promotes)

## SECONDARY APPLICATIONS

Abdominal cramps
Coughs
Earache
Gout
Leprosy
Mucus
Phlegm (expels)
Pneumonia
Sunstroke
Tuberculosis
Uterus

Convulsions
Delirium
Flu
Headaches, migraine
Measles
Nausea
Pleurisy
Smallpox
Toothache
Ulcers
Vertigo

# PEPPERMINT (*Mentha piperita*)

*PART USED:* LEAVES

Peppermint is good for many remedies and is useful to have in the house. It contains a warming oil that is effective as a nerve stimulant. The oil brings oxygen into the blood stream and works to clean and strengthen the entire body. Peppermint also acts as a sedative on the stomach and helps strengthen the bowels. It is useful for bowel problems, convulsions and spasms in children. It works on the salivary glands to aid in digestion. It is useful for chills and colds, and can be used for many other ailments. Peppermint contains vitamins A and C, magnesium, potassium, inositol, niacin, copper, iodine, silicon, iron and sulphur.

## PRIMARY APPLICATIONS

| | |
|---|---|
| Appetite | Colds |
| Colic | Digestion |
| Fever | Gas |
| Headaches | Heartburn |
| Shock | |

## SECONDARY APPLICATIONS

| | |
|---|---|
| Bowel spasms | Chills |
| Cholera | Constipation |
| Convulsions | Cramps, stomach |
| Depression, mental | Dizziness |
| Fainting | Flu |
| Heart | Hysteria |
| Insomnia | Measles |
| Menstruation pain | Morning sickness |
| Mouthwash | Nausea |
| Nerves | Neuralgia |
| Nightmares | Seasickness |
| Stomach spasms | Vomiting |

# PERIWINKLE (*Vinca major; Vinca minor*)

PARTS USED: ENTIRE PLANT

Periwinkle has been reported by British physicians to contain a substance called vinblastine sulphate. This substance has shown promise in treating choriocarcinoma and Hodgkin's disease. This herb is under further research for use with other types of cancer. Periwinkle is also considered a good binder and, when chewed, works to stop bleeding of the nose or mouth. It also helps with female problems.

PRIMARY APPLICATIONS

Cancer
Nervousness

Diabetes
Ulcers

SECONDARY APPLICATIONS

Bleeding
Constipation, chronic
Dandruff, external
Fits
Hysteria
Mucus
Skin disorders
Toothache

Congestion
Cramps
Diarrhea, chronic
Hemorrhages, internal
Leukemia
Nightmares
Sores
Wounds

# PLANTAIN (*Plantago major*)

PARTS USED: LEAVES AND SEEDS

Plantain will neutralize stomach acids and normalize all stomach secretions. The fresh juice has been used in mild stomach ulcers. Plantain tea clears the head and ears of mucus. The tea is also useful in treating chronic lung problems in children. The herb is known to neutralize poisons. The leaves, when applied to a bleeding surface, will stop hemorrhaging. The seeds are related to psyllium seeds and can be used in the same way. Plantain is rich in vitamins C, K and T, calcium, potassium, and sulphur. It also has a high content of trace minerals.

## PRIMARY APPLICATIONS

| | |
|---|---|
| Bedwetting | Bladder infections |
| Blood poisoning | Diarrhea |
| Kidney | Neuralgia |
| Snake bites | Sores |

## SECONDARY APPLICATIONS

| | |
|---|---|
| Bronchitis | Burns |
| Coughs | Cuts |
| Dropsy | Dysentery |
| Epilepsy | Eyes, sore |
| Fevers, intermittent | Gas |
| Hemorrhages, external | Hemorrhoids |
| Infections | Insect bites |
| Jaundice | Leucorrhea |
| Menstruation, excessive | Respiratory problems |
| Scalds | Scrofula |
| Skin problems | Stings |

# PLEURISY ROOT (Asclepias tuberosa)

## PART USED: ROOT

Pleurisy root is an effective expectorant. It helps expel phlegm from bronchial and nasal passages. It is a gentle tonic for stomach pain caused by gas, indigestion and dysentery. As the name implies, this herb is valuable in treating pleurisy, helping relieve the pain and difficulty of breathing. Pleurisy root is not recommended for children.

## PRIMARY APPLICATIONS

| | |
|---|---|
| Asthma, spasmodic | Bronchitis |
| Dysentery, acute | Emphysema |
| Fevers | Lung problems |
| Pleurisy | Pneumonia |

## SECONDARY APPLICATIONS

| | |
|---|---|
| Contagious diseases | Croup |
| Flu | Kidneys |
| Measles | Mucus |
| Perspiration | Poisoning |
| Rheumatism, acute | Scarlet fever |
| Tuberculosis | Typhus |

# POKEWEED (*Phytolacca americana*)

## PARTS USED: ROOT AND YOUNG SHOOTS

Pokeweed is an excellent remedy for enlarged glands (lymphatic, spleen and thyroid), hardening of the liver, and reduced biliary flow. It stimulates metabolism and is a useful medication for the undernourished. It reduces inflammation, so it is good for rheumatism, tonsillitis, laryngitis and mumps. Pokeweed, applied as a powdered root poultice, has traditionally been used by Native Americans as a cure for surface cancers and skin eruptions. It is now widely used as a salve to treat scabies, acne and fungal infections, and as a poultice for abscesses. Pokeweed contains steroids resembling cortisone, making it useful in treating psoriasis and other skin conditions, rheumatism, and slow-healing wounds. Pokeweed should be used sparingly and by one trained in herbs. It contains vitamins A and C, calcium, iron, and phosphorus.

PRIMARY APPLICATIONS

| | |
|---|---|
| Arthritis | Blood purifier |
| Glands | Inflammation |
| Pain | Rheumatism |

SECONDARY APPLICATIONS

| | |
|---|---|
| Cancer | Catarrh, chronic |
| Goiter | Laryngitis |
| Laxative | Lymphs |
| Mumps | Respiratory problems |
| Scrofula | Skin diseases |
| Tonsillitis | |

# PRICKLY ASH  *(Xanthoxylum fraxineum)*

PART USED: BARK

*P*rickly ash is a stimulant herb that increases circulation throughout the body. It is beneficial as a remedy for cold extremities and joints, rheumatism, arthritis, lethargy, and wounds that are slow to heal. Prickly ash can be applied externally as a poultice to help dry up and heal wounds. The powdered bark has been chewed for relief of toothache. Prickly ash helps increase the flow of saliva and moistens a dry tongue (conditions which often accompany liver malfunctions).

PRIMARY APPLICATIONS

| | |
|---|---|
| Circulation, poor | Fever |
| Sores, Mouth | Ulcers |
| Wounds | |

SECONDARY APPLICATIONS

| | |
|---|---|
| Arthritis | Asthma |
| Blood purifier | Cholera |

| | |
|---|---|
| Colic | Cramps |
| Digestion, weak | Diarrhea |
| Gas | Lethargy |
| Liver problems | Paralysis |
| Rheumatism, chronic | Syphilis |

# PSYLLIUM (*Plantago ovata*)

*PART USED:* SEEDS

*P*syllium is considered an excellent colon and intestine cleanser. It does not irritate the mucous membranes of the intestines, but strengthens the tissues and restores tone. It lubricates as well as heals the intestines and colon. It is said to be a good remedy for autointoxication—the cause of many diseases—by cleansing the intestines and removing toxins.

## PRIMARY APPLICATIONS

| | |
|---|---|
| Colon blockage | Constipation |
| Diverticulitis | |

## SECONDARY APPLICATIONS

| | |
|---|---|
| Colitis | Dysentery |
| Gonorrhea | Hemorrhage |
| Intestinal tract | Ulcers |
| Urinary tract | |

# PYGEUM (*Prunus africana*)

*PART USED:* BARK

*P*ygeum is commonly partnered with saw palmetto and found in herbal combinations used for the prostate gland. This is because it contains compounds known for their ability to reduce inflammation of the prostate. Many European physicians prescribe pygeum for benign prostatic hyperplasia which can cause urination problems. It is also used as a preventive measure for prostate health.

## PRIMARY APPLICATIONS

Prostate gland enlargement    Prostate health
Urination problems

## SECONDARY APPLICATIONS

Circulation    Energy
Fatigue    Impotency

# QUASSIA (Picrasma amara)

PART USED: BARK

Quassia is a great healer of the sick. It is a powerful herb and if taken in excess can be an emetic, irritant, depressant, and produce nausea. But, if taken in small doses, it is a speedy cure. It is considered one of the best remedies for noxious substances found in the alimentary canal that result from the digestion process. It is also a good tonic to help run down systems. Quassia is said to be a good remedy to destroy the taste for strong drink. It is also beneficial to the eyes because it keeps the liver in good working condition. Quassia contains calcium, sodium, and potassium.

## PRIMARY APPLICATIONS

Appetite, stimulant    Digestion
Fevers    Tonic

## SECONDARY APPLICATIONS

Alcoholism    Constipation
Dandruff, external    Dyspepsia
Pinworms (through enema)    Rheumatism

# QUEEN OF THE MEADOW
*(Eupatorium purpureum)*
PART USED: *LEAVES*

Queen of the meadow is useful for all ills of the joints, especially joint pains caused by uric acid deposits. It is also used for strains, sprains, and pulled ligaments and tendons. This herb is well known for its usefulness with rheumatism, dropsy, kidney and gallstones. It is useful in treating water retention and has been used for chronic urinary problems, gout and cystitis. Queen of the meadow contains vitamins C and D.

## PRIMARY APPLICATIONS

| | |
|---|---|
| Bursitis | Gallstones |
| Kidney infections | Kidney stones |
| Neuralgia | Rheumatism |
| Ringworm | Urinary problems |
| Water retention | |

## SECONDARY APPLICATIONS

| | |
|---|---|
| Bladder infections | Diabetes |
| Gout | Headaches |
| Lumbago | Nerve problems |
| Prostate | Typhus |

# RED CLOVER *(Trifolium pratense)*

PART USED: *FLOWER*

Red clover is useful as a tonic for the nerves and as a sedative for nervous exhaustion. It is a very useful herb for children because of its mild alterative properties, as well as its mild sedative effect. It is useful as a cough syrup when mixed with honey and water. It is also good for weak lungs, wheezing, bronchitis, and for lack of vitality. Red clover is a valuable herb for treating wasting diseases (especially rickets), spasmodic affections, and whooping cough. It is being researched as a possible antidote to cancer. Native Americans have long used the plant for sore eyes and burns. Red clover is a valuable dietary supplement because it supplies vitamin A and is high in iron, magnesium, calcium and copper. It also contains vitamins C, F, P and B-complex, some selenium, cobalt, nickel, manganese, sodium, and tin.

## PRIMARY APPLICATIONS

| | |
|---|---|
| Blood purifier | Bronchitis |
| Cancer | Nerves |
| Spasms | Toxins |

## SECONDARY APPLICATIONS

| | |
|---|---|
| Acne | Arthritis |
| Appetite | Athletes' foot poultice |
| Boils | Burns |
| Childhood diseases | Coughs |
| Eyewash | Flu |
| Leprosy | Liver problems |
| Psoriasis | Rheumatism |
| Skin diseases | Sores |
| Syphilis | Tumors |
| Ulcers | Urinary problems |

# RED RASPBERRY (*Rubus idaeus*)

## PART USED: LEAVES

Red raspberry is one of the most renowned herbs used by women, especially during pregnancy. It contains nutrients that help to strengthen the uterus wall, reduce nausea, prevent hemorrhage, and reduce pain of childbirth. Red raspberry helps reduce false labor pains common in some pregnancies. It also helps enrich the colostrum found in breast milk. Drinking the tea will relieve painful menstruation and aid the blood flow. If your flow is too heavy, red raspberry tea will help it decrease gradually. Drinking the tea after childbirth will help decrease uterine swelling and cut down on post-partum bleeding. Besides being good for women, red raspberry is a wonderful herb for children to use in case of colds, diarrhea, colic and fevers. It is also a good remedy for infants who suffer from dysentery and diarrhea. Red raspberry contains vitamins A, C, D, E, G, F, and B. It is rich in iron and calcium and contains phosphorus and manganese.

## PRIMARY APPLICATIONS

| | |
|---|---|
| Afterpains | Bowel problems |
| Childbirth | Diarrhea |
| Female organs | Fevers |
| Flu | Morning sickness |
| Mouth sores | Nausea |
| Pregnancy | Vomiting |

## SECONDARY APPLICATIONS

| | |
|---|---|
| Bronchitis | Canker sores |
| Cholera | Colds |
| Constipation | Diabetes |
| Digestion | Dysentery |
| Eye wash | Hemorrhoids |
| Lactation | Leucorrhea |
| Measles | Menstruation |
| Nervousness | Stomach |
| Teething | Throat, sore |
| Urinary problems | Uterus, prolapsed |

# REDMOND CLAY (*Montmorillonite*)

*PART USED: CLAY*

Redmond clay is used externally for skin problems. It is good to have around for stings, bug bites and for expelling worms from the intestinal tract. It also helps heal muscle sprains and wounds. It can be used for fevers and will quickly absorb poisons in the stomach if taken with a glass of water.

## PRIMARY APPLICATIONS

Bee stings                      Skin problems

## SECONDARY APPLICATIONS

Acne                            Bug bites
Poisoning, internal             Worms

# REISHI

*PARTS USED: BODY AND STEM*

Reishi mushroom has been found to help in stimulating and strengthening the immune system. For this reason it may be beneficial for conditions such as cancer, tumors, AIDS, chronic fatigue syndrome, and allergies. It may also help lower cholesterol and triglyceride levels. It has been used to strengthen the heart and cardiovascular system. Reishi has also been used successfully to alleviate insomnia and calm the nervous system. It aids in relieving stress and allowing for relaxation.

## PRIMARY APPLICATIONS

Aids                            Allergies
Fatigue                         Heart problems
Insomnia

## SECONDARY APPLICATIONS

Blood Pressure
Cardiovascular System
Diabetes
Nervousness

Cancer
Cholesterol
Longevity

# RHUBARB *(Rheum palmatum)*

*PART USED: ROOT*

Rhubarb is a mildly stimulating tonic for the liver, gall ducts and mucous membranes in the intestines. It acts as a laxative, cleansing intestinal irritants and checking diarrhea with its astringent action. Rhubarb is useful when the stomach is weak and the bowels are relaxed because it acts as a gentle cathartic. It is very useful in toxic blood conditions caused by excessive intake of meat. Rhubarb contains vitamins A, C and B-complex, sodium, potassium, some iron, sulphur, phosphorus, cobalt, nickel and tin. It is high in calcium.

## PRIMARY APPLICATIONS

Colon
Liver problems

Diarrhea

## SECONDARY APPLICATIONS

Anemia
Constipation
Dysentery
Gallbladder
Stomach

Colitis
Digestion aids
Jaundice
Headaches

# ROSE HIPS *(Rosa species)*

*PART USED:* FRUIT

Rose hips are an excellent source of vitamin C. They contain substantially more vitamin C than citrus and are also rich in vitamins A, E and rutin. The use of hips is recommended to help expel kidney stones. They are very nourishing to the skin and help prevent and reduce infections. Rose hips are very high in vitamins A, B-complex, C, E and also contain vitamins D and P, organic iron, sodium, potassium, sulphur, silica, and niacin. They are a good source of natural fruit sugar.

## PRIMARY APPLICATIONS

Blood purifier
Colds
Infections

Cancer
Flu
Throat, sore

## SECONDARY APPLICATIONS

Arteriosclerosis
Bruises
Contagious diseases
Dizziness
Fever
Kidney stones
Psoriasis

Bites
Circulation
Cramps
Earaches
Headaches
Mouth sores
Stings

# ROSEMARY *(Rosmarinus officinalis)*

*PART USED:* LEAVES

Rosemary is a strong stimulant that works mainly on the circulatory system and the pelvic region. It is one of the few proven heart tonics that is not a drastic drug. It is also a treatment for high blood pressure. Rosemary is used externally for wounds of all kinds, including bites and stings. It is excellent for various female ailments—it helps regulate menses and should be thought of when there are uterus pains followed by hemorrhage. It is a good tonic for the reproductive organs. Rosemary tea will help relieve hysterical depression and is very good for headaches caused by nerves because it stimulates the nervous system. In fact, it is considered one of the most powerful natural remedies to strengthen the nervous system.

Rosemary can be taken in the early states of colds and flu as a warm infusion, and may be used as a cooling tea when there is restlessness, nervousness, and insomnia. Rosemary, sage, and vervain in equal parts make an antiseptic drink for fevers. Rosemary has also been known for preventing premature baldness and stimulating increased activity of the "hair-bulbs." This herb is high in calcium. It contains vitamins A and C, iron, magnesium, phosphorus, potassium, sodium and zinc.

## PRIMARY APPLICATIONS

| | |
|---|---|
| Halitosis | Headaches, migraine |
| Heart tonic | Stomach disorder |

## SECONDARY APPLICATIONS

| | |
|---|---|
| Baldness | Circulation |
| Convulsions | Digestion |
| Dropsy | Eczema |
| Eye wash | Female problems |
| Gallbladder | Gas |
| Hair (stimulates) | High blood pressure |
| Hysteria | Liver |
| Memory | Menstruation |
| Nervousness | Prostate |
| Spasms | Sores, open |
| Stings, external | Wounds |

# RUE *(Ruta graveolens)*

PARTS USED: *ENTIRE PLANT*

Rue can be used for a variety of ailments. It has the ability to expel poisons from the body and has been used for snake, scorpion, spider and jellyfish bites. Rue has also been found very effective in preserving sight by strengthening the ocular muscles. Rue helps remove deposits that are liable to form with age in the tendons and joints, especially in the wrist. Rue contains large amounts of rutin (vitamin P) which is known for its ability to strengthen capillaries and veins. The U.S. Department of Agriculture has found that rutin is very effective in treating high blood pressure and also helps to harden the bones and teeth. Because of its emetic properties, rue should not be used before meals and should not be taken by pregnant women.

## PRIMARY APPLICATIONS

| | |
|---|---|
| Blood pressure, high | Cramps |
| Hypertension | Hysteria |
| Muscles, strained | Neuralgia |
| Nervous disorder | Sciatica |
| Tendons, strained | Trauma |

## SECONDARY APPLICATIONS

| | |
|---|---|
| Arteriosclerosis | Bruising, easy |
| Circulation, poor | Colic |
| Convulsions | Coughs |
| Croup, spasmodic | Earaches |
| Eye ailments | Epilepsy |
| Female problems | Insanity |
| Malaria | Metabolism (improves) |
| Nosebleeds, chronic | Poisons (antidote for) |
| Typhoid | Varicose veins |
| Whooping cough | Worms |

# SAFFLOWER (*Carthamus tinctorius*)

## PART USED: FLOWERS

Safflower is a good remedy for jaundice and other liver and gallbladder problems. It can be used for fevers and various other childhood complaints. It also has the ability to remove hard phlegm from the body, clear the lungs and help in pulmonary tuberculosis. Safflower has gained popularity in the past few years because of the unsaturated oil found in its seeds. Safflower contains vitamin K.

### PRIMARY APPLICATIONS

| | |
|---|---|
| Delirium | Digestion |
| Fevers | Gout |
| Jaundice | Liver |
| Phlegm | Sweating |
| Uric acid | Urinary problems |

### SECONDARY APPLICATIONS

| | |
|---|---|
| Boils, external | Chicken pox |
| Gallbladder | Gout |
| Heart (strengthens) | Hysteria |
| Measles | Menstruation |
| Mumps | Poison ivy |
| Sweating | Tuberculosis |

# SAFFRON (*Crocus satirus*)

## PART USED: FLOWERS

Saffron soothes the membranes of the stomach and colon. It helps reduce cholesterol levels by neutralizing the build-up of uric acid in the body. It has been known to prevent heart disease.

In Valencia, a region in Spain, saffron is eaten daily and little heart disease exists there. Saffron contains vitamins A and B12. It also has potassium, some calcium, phosphorus, sodium, and lactic acid.

## PRIMARY APPLICATIONS

| | |
|---|---|
| Fevers | Gout |
| Measles | Rheumatism |
| Scarlet fever | |

## SECONDARY APPLICATIONS

| | |
|---|---|
| Arthritis | Bronchitis |
| Coughs | Digestion |
| Gas | Headaches |
| Heartburn | Hyperglycemia |
| Hypoglycemia | Insomnia |
| Jaundice | Menstruation |
| Psoriasis | Skin diseases |
| Stomach disorders | Ulcers, internal |
| Uterine hemorrhages | Water retention |

# SAGE (Salvia officinalis)

## PART USED: LEAVES

Sage is used for excessive mucus discharge, nasal drip, indurated sores and excessive secretions of saliva. This herb was traditionally used as a staple in the home and was thought to prolong life. It was used as a lotion to heal sores and other skin eruptions. The fresh leaves were also chewed as a remedy for infections of the mouth and throat. Sage is beneficial for mental exhaustion and for increasing the ability to concentrate. It improves memory and has been used to cure some types of insanity. Sage contains vitamins A, C, and vitamin B-complex, sulphur, silicon, phosphorus, and sodium. It is high in calcium and potassium.

## PRIMARY APPLICATIONS

Coughs
Fevers
Memory (improves)
Nausea
Throat, sore

Digestion
Gums, sore
Mouth sores
Nerves

## SECONDARY APPLICATIONS

Brain, (stimulates)
Blood infections
Diarrhea
Flu
Hair growth
Lactation (stops)
Lung congestion
Palsy
Phlegm
Snake bites
Tonsillitis
Worms`

Bladder infection
Colds
Dysentery
Gravel
Headaches
Laryngitis
Night sweats
Parasites
Sinus congestion
Teeth cleanser
Ulcers
Yeast Infections

# ST. JOHN'S WORT

*(Hypericum perforatum)*
PARTS USED: ENTIRE PLANT

St. John's wort contains hypericin, a compound being researched for use in treating AIDS, cancer and various viruses. Recent research has also shown St. John's wort to be very effective in treating mild to moderate depression. It is an effective remedy for headaches accompanied by excitability, hysteria and neuralgia, especially when such symptoms occur during menopause. This herb is helpful for obstructions of phlegm in the chest and lungs and has been known to eliminate all signs of bronchitis. It is useful in healing wounds, even dirty, septic ones. St. John's wort helps reduce mild pain in the stomach, intestines and gallbladder.

## PRIMARY APPLICATIONS

Depression
Antiviral therapy
Afterpains
Skin problems

AIDS
Cancer therapy
Bronchitis

## SECONDARY APPLICATIONS

Appetite
Bleeding (internal)
Boils
Diarrhea
Hemorrhaging
Insomnia
Lung congestion
Menopause
Nervousness
Tumors
Urine, suppressed

Bites, insect
Blood purifier
Breasts, caked
Dysentery
Hysteria
Jaundice
Melancholy
Menstruation, painful
Spasms
Ulcers
Uterine

# SARSAPARILLA (*Smilax ornata*)

## PART USED: ROOT

Sarsaparilla is a valuable herb used in glandular balance formulas. It contains both testosterone and progesterone and its stimulating properties are noted for increasing metabolic rate. It increases circulation to rheumatic joints and stimulates breathing in problems of congestion. Sarsaparilla contains vitamins A, C, D and B-complex. It also has iron, manganese, sodium, silicon, sulphur, copper, zinc, and iodine.

## PRIMARY APPLICATIONS

Blood purifier          Gas
Joint aches             Hormones
Skin diseases

## SECONDARY APPLICATIONS

Age spots               Colds
Dropsy                  Eyes, sore
Fevers                  Gout
Menopause               Physical debility
Psoriasis               Rheumatism, chronic
Ring worm               Sexual impotence
Scrofula                Skin parasites
Sores                   Venereal diseases

# SASSAFRAS (Sassafras officinale)

### PART USED: ROOT BARK

Sassafras stimulates the liver to clear toxins from the system, making it a good tonic, especially after childbirth. It has been used as a pain reliever and also to treat venereal diseases. Native Americans used an infusion of sassafras roots to bring down a fever. Sassafras and burdock are excellent together as an appetite-control tonic. The ingredients of these herbs aid the pituitary gland in releasing an ample supply of protein, which helps adjust hormone balance in the body.

## PRIMARY APPLICATIONS

Acne                    Blood purifier
Obesity                 Psoriasis
Skin diseases           Water retention

## SECONDARY APPLICATIONS

| | |
|---|---|
| Afterpains | Bladder problems |
| Boils | Bronchitis |
| Colic | Cramps, stomach |
| Diarrhea | Gas |
| Kidney problems | Perspiration, increases |
| Poison ivy and oak | Rheumatism |
| Spasms | Varicose ulcers |

# SAW PALMETTO (*Serenoa serrulata*)

## PART USED: FRUIT

Saw palmetto is recommended for wasting diseases because it effects glandular tissues. It is also useful for diseases of the reproductive glands. The crushed root was used by Native Americans for sore breasts, and has been said to increase the size of small breasts. Saw palmetto is used to soothe mucous membranes of the throat and nose, and is considered a tonic for chronic bronchitis and lung asthma. This herb contains vitamin A.

## PRIMARY APPLICATIONS

| | |
|---|---|
| Digestion | Glands |
| Reproductive organs | Sex stimulant |
| Weight (increases) | |

## SECONDARY APPLICATIONS

| | |
|---|---|
| Asthma | Bladder diseases |
| Bronchitis, chronic | Catarrhal problems |
| Colds, head | Kidney diseases |
| Lung congestion | Mucus (excess) |
| Nerves | Urinary problems |

# SCHIZANDRA (Schisandra chinensis)

## PART USED: BERRIES

Schizandra is capable of increasing the body's immune system and protecting against stress. It is an adaptogen herb that increases the energy supply to cells in the brain, muscles, liver, kidneys and nerves. It protects against free radical damage and helps to balance body functions. It contains properties which nourish the veins and improve vision. It can also protect against radiation, counteract effects of sugar, boost stamina, normalize blood sugar and pressure, and protect against infections. Schizandra is high in vitamin C, magnesium, phosphorus, and contains calcium, iron, potassium, selenium, silicon and sodium.

## PRIMARY APPLICATIONS

| | |
|---|---|
| Energy, increases | Mental alertness |
| Nervous disorder | Stress |

## SECONDARY APPLICATIONS

| | |
|---|---|
| Atherosclerosis | Insomnia |
| Blood pressure, normalizes | Coughs |
| Digestive problems | Fatigue |
| Gastritis, chronic | Hepatitis |
| Kidney problems | Lung problems |
| Motion sickness | Radiation |
| Uterine problems | Vision, improves |

# SKULLCAP (Scutellaria lateriflora)

## PARTS USED: ENTIRE PLANT

Skullcap is called "a food for the nerves." It supports and strengthens the nerves and so gives immediate relief from diseases stemming from nervous affections and debility. Skullcap has traditionally been used to cure infertility. It is also said to regulate undue sexual desires. Mixed with pennyroyal this herb has been used successfully as a remedy for cramps and severe pain caused by suppressed menstruation due to colds. Skullcap is high in calcium, potassium, and magnesium. It also contains vitamins C, E, iron and zinc.

## PRIMARY APPLICATIONS

| | |
|---|---|
| Convulsions | Epilepsy |
| Fevers (reduces) | High blood pressure |
| Infertility | Insomnia |
| Nerves | Restlessness |

## SECONDARY APPLICATIONS

| | |
|---|---|
| Aches | Alcoholism |
| Blood pressure | Childhood diseases |
| Delirium | Drug withdrawal |
| Headaches | Hypertension |
| Hysteria | Hypoglycemia |
| Palsy | Parkinson's disease |
| Poisonous bites | Rabies |
| Rheumatism | Spinal meningitis |
| St. Vitus' dance | Thyroid problems |
| Tremors | Urinary |

# SENEGA *(Polygala senega)*

## PART USED: ROOT

Senega is used as an expectorant in respiratory problems. It is useful in the second stage of acute bronchial catarrh and pneumonia. It increases secretions and circulation and is useful when there is prostration from blood poisoning, small pox, asthma, and diseases of the lungs. It has been said to be an excellent antidote for many poisons. Senega contains magnesium, iron, tin, lead and aluminum in small amounts.

## PRIMARY APPLICATIONS

| | |
|---|---|
| Asthma | Bronchitis, chronic |
| Croup | Lung congestion |
| Mucus (in tissues) | Pneumonia |
| Snakebites | |

## SECONDARY APPLICATIONS

| | |
|---|---|
| Blood poisoning | Drugs, (side effects) |
| Pleurisy | Rheumatism |

# SENNA (*Cassia acutifolia*)

## PARTS USED: LEAVES AND PODS

Senna is a very useful laxative. It increases the intestinal peristaltic movements and has a strong effect on the entire intestinal tract, especially the colon. It should always be taken with carminative herbs such as ginger or fennel to prevent bowel cramps. It should not be used in cases of inflammation of the stomach. Senna is a very useful herb to cleanse the system during fasting and in case of fever. It tones and restores the digestive system as it thoroughly cleanses.

## PRIMARY APPLICATIONS

| | |
|---|---|
| Constipation | Jaundice |

## SECONDARY APPLICATIONS

| | |
|---|---|
| Bad breath | Biliousness |
| Colic | Gallstones |

| | |
|---|---|
| Gout | Menstruation |
| Obesity | Pimples |
| Rheumatism | Skin diseases |
| Sores, mouth | Worms |

# SHEPHERD'S PURSE

*(Capsella bursa-pastoris)*
PARTS USED: *ENTIRE PLANT*

Shepherd's purse is used for cases of hemorrhaging after childbirth, excessive menstruation, and internal bleeding in the lungs and colon. It helps to constrict the blood vessels and is used to regulate blood pressure and heart action. It acts as a stimulant and tonic for catarrh of the urinary tract (indicated by mucus in the urine). Shepherd's purse is high in vitamin C and contains vitamins E and K. It also has iron, magnesium, calcium, potassium, tin, zinc, sodium, and sulphur.

## PRIMARY APPLICATIONS

| | |
|---|---|
| Bleeding | Blood pressure |
| Bloody urine | Ear ailments |
| Menstruation, painful | |

## SECONDARY APPLICATIONS

| | |
|---|---|
| Arteriosclerosis | Bowels |
| Constipation | Diarrhea |
| Heart | Hemorrhage |
| Kidney problems | Lumbago |
| Uterus | Vagina |
| Water retention | |

# SHIITAKE (*Lentinus edodes*)

*PARTS USED: STEM AND CAP*

Shiitake mushroom is an immune system stimulant and strengthener. It is used to prevent cancer and other immune-related conditions. It also helps with viral and bacterial infections. Shiitake is used throughout Asia to treat many problems such as high blood pressure, heart disease and cholesterol.

## PRIMARY APPLICATIONS

Immune system

## SECONDARY APPLICATIONS

Blood Pressure                    Cancer
Cholesterol                       Infections
Longevity

# SLIPPERY ELM (*Ulmus fulva*)

*PARTS USED: INNER BARK*

Slippery elm has the ability to neutralize stomach acidity and to absorb gases. It aids in the digestion of milk. This herb also acts as a buffer against irritations and inflammations of the mucous membranes. It has the ability to remove mucus with stronger force than other herbs. Slippery elm assists the adrenal glands by helping boost the output of cortin hormone. This helps send a stream of blood-building substances through the system. Slippery elm draws out impurities and heals all parts of the body. It is also used whenever there is difficulty holding and digesting food. Slippery elm contains vitamins E, F, K and P. It also contains iron, sodium, calcium, selenium, iodine, copper, zinc and some potassium and phosphorus.

## PRIMARY APPLICATIONS

| | |
|---|---|
| Asthma | Bronchitis |
| Burns | Colitis |
| Colon | Coughs |
| Diaper rash | Diarrhea |
| Digestion | Lung problems |

## SECONDARY APPLICATIONS

| | |
|---|---|
| Appendicitis | Bladder problems |
| Boils | Bowels |
| Cancer | Constipation |
| Croup | Female problems |
| Hemorrhoids | Herpes |
| Inflammations | Laxative |
| Pain | Phlegm |
| Poison ivy, external | Sores |
| Syphilis | Throat, sore |
| Tuberculosis | Tumors |
| Ulcers | Urinary problems |
| Vaginal irritations | Wound |

# SPEARMINT (*Mentha viridis*)

## PART USED: LEAVES

Spearmint is a valuable herb that even the sickest person can tolerate because it has no toxicity. It is excellent for stopping vomiting during pregnancy. The oil in spearmint leaves works on the salivary glands to aid in digestion. It stimulates gastric secretion and is credited with an action of biliary secretion. It is a gentle and effective remedy for babies with colic. Spearmint is an excellent source of vitamins C and A. It also contains B-complex, calcium, sulphur, iron, iodine, magnesium and potassium.

## PRIMARY APPLICATIONS

| | |
|---|---|
| Colds | Colic |
| Flu | Gas |
| Nausea | Vomiting |

## SECONDARY APPLICATIONS

| | |
|---|---|
| Bladder inflammation | Chills |
| Cramps | Dizziness |
| Dropsy | Fever |
| Hysteria | Indigestion |
| Kidney inflammation | Spasms |
| Kidney stones | Urine, suppressed |

# SPIKENARD *(Aralia racemosa)*

## PART USED: ROOT

Spikenard tea has traditionally been given to women before labor to make childbirth easier and to help shorten the ordeal. It is also useful for reducing uric acid build-up and has been combined with other herbs to purify and build the blood. Spikenard has a slight expectorant effect and is useful in cough syrups, along with other herbs. The properties of this herb are very close to ginseng. The Russians use the roots as a general tonic and stimulant, especially for physical and mental exhaustion.

## PRIMARY APPLICATIONS

| | |
|---|---|
| Asthma | Childbirth |
| Cough | Rheumatism |

## SECONDARY APPLICATIONS

| | |
|---|---|
| Backache | Blood purifier |
| Chest pains | Diarrhea |
| Hay fever | Hemorrhoids |

Inflammation
Lung congestion

Venereal diseases
Skin problems

# SPIRULINA *(Spirulina pratensis)*

*PARTS USED: ENTIRE PLANT*

Spirulina is a natural food supplement used in weight control diets. It provides nutrients that satisfy hunger which occurs when the body is not getting enough essential nutrition. It is considered one of nature's whole foods and is easily digestible. It strengthens the body and provides nutrients when the body is weak, either after an acute illness or during a chronic disease. Spirulina is rich in protein, chlorophyll and essential fatty acids. It is high in A and B vitamins, including B12. It is also high in iron, magnesium and phosphorus and contains calcium, potassium, sodium, vitamin C and E. It contains almost all nutrients required by the body.

*PRIMARY APPLICATIONS*

Blood builder
Food supplement

Chronic diseases
Tonic

*SECONDARY APPLICATIONS*

Anemia
Blood pressure, regulates
Goiter
Hypoglycemia

Appetite suppressant
Diets
Gout
Skin problems

# STEVIA *(Stevia rebaudiana)*

*PART USED: LEAVES*

Stevia is a natural sweetener, 30 to 100 times sweeter than sugar. Small amounts go a long way and, unlike other sugar substitutes, there is no after-taste. Research in Japan has found stevia to be safe and nontoxic so it is used in soy sauce, chewing gum and mouthwash. It is non-fattening and can be used on cereals and in herbal teas. Stevia is high in chromium, (which helps to establish blood sugar), manganese, potassium, selenium, silicon, sodium and vitamin A. It also contains iron, niacin, phosphorus, riboflavin, thiamine, vitamin C, and zinc.

### PRIMARY APPLICATIONS

| | |
|---|---|
| Diabetes | Food cravings |
| Obesity | Tobacco cravings |
| Sugar substitute | |

### SECONDARY APPLICATIONS

| | |
|---|---|
| Addictions | Hypertension |
| Hypoglycemia | |

# SQUAW VINE (*Mitchella repens*)

### PART USED: ENTIRE PLANT

Squaw vine is especially helpful in childbirth. It strengthens the uterus for a safe and effective childbirth. It is called a uterine tonic because it relieves congestion of the uterus and ovaries. It also helps restore menstrual function. Squaw vine contains antiseptic properties, which makes it ideal for any kind of vaginal infection. It is also beneficial as a natural sedative on the nerves. It is best used with other herbs, such as red raspberry.

### PRIMARY APPLICATIONS

| | |
|---|---|
| Childbirth, eases | Lactation |
| Menstruation | Uterine disorders |

SECONDARY APPLICATIONS

| | |
|---|---|
| Bites, snake | Diarrhea |
| Eyes, sore | Gonorrhea |
| Hemorrhoids | Nerves |
| Insomnia | Skin problems |
| Syphilis | Urinary problems |
| Varicose veins | Water retention |

# STILLINGIA  (*Stillingia ligustina*)

PART USED: ROOT

Stillingia is one of the most powerful herb alternatives known. It is an effective glandular stimulant, as well as an activator for the liver. It is said to be valuable for ridding the system of toxic drugs caused by chemotherapy. It should be used with caution and is used best in combination with other herbs.

PRIMARY APPLICATIONS

| | |
|---|---|
| Acne | Blood purifier |
| Eczema | Liver problems |
| Respiratory problems | Skin problems |
| Syphilis | |

SECONDARY APPLICATIONS

| | |
|---|---|
| Bronchitis | Constipation |
| Throat, sore | Urinary problems |

# STRAWBERRY  (*Fragaria vesca*)

PART USED: LEAVES

Strawberry aids in the overall health of the body. It acts as a cleanser for the stomach and is useful for bowel troubles. The roots are especially useful for obstinate dysentery. It has been used for eczema, externally and internally. Discolored teeth or teeth encrusted with tarter can be cleaned with strawberry juice. Strawberry leaves are rich in iron and contain vitamins A, C, B-complex, calcium, phosphorus, and potassium. This herb is safe and useful for children.

## PRIMARY APPLICATIONS

| | |
|---|---|
| Blood purifier | Diarrhea |
| Eczema | Intestines |
| Miscarriage (prevents) | Stomach, cleans |

## SECONDARY APPLICATIONS

| | |
|---|---|
| Acne | Bowel problems |
| Dysentery | Fevers |
| High blood pressure (lowers) | Jaundice |
| Lactation | Nerves |
| Vomiting | |

# SUMA (Pfaffia paniculata)

## PART USED: BARK AND ROOT

Suma is an adaptogen herb, one used to heal and prevent disease. It is a nutrient that helps protect the immune system, relieves stress and helps the body to adapt to many environmental and psychological stresses. It is an herb that benefits both men and women because it restores sexual function, protects against viral infections and benefits cancer victims. Research in Japan has discovered a unique chemical in suma that tends to inhibit tumor cell growth. Suma also contains allantoin (also found in comfrey), a compound known to promote the healing of wounds and new cell growth. Another benefit of this herb is that it contains two plant hormones, sitosterol and stipmasterol, found to be beneficial to human metabolism by increasing circulation and decreasing high blood cholesterol levels. Sitosterol enhances the body's natural production of estrogen when stores are depleted. It works to prevent the random release of free radicals. Portuguese call suma "para todo" meaning "for everything"—a good indication of all this herb is capable of. Suma contains germanium, iron and magnesium.

## PRIMARY APPLICATIONS

| | |
|---|---|
| Circulation problems | Cholesterol |
| Chronic diseases | Fatigue |
| Hormone regulator | Immune system |
| Stress | Tonic |

## SECONDARY APPLICATIONS

| | |
|---|---|
| Anemia | Arthritis |
| Balance hormones | Bronchitis |
| Cancer | Colds |
| Diabetes | Energy booster |
| Heart disease | Hypoglycemia |
| Joint diseases | Menopause systems |
| Premenstrual problems | Osteomelitis |
| Osteoporosis | Skin problems |
| Strokes | Tumors |

# TAHEEBO (SEE PAU D'ARCO)

# TEA TREE OIL (Meleleuca alternifolia)

PART USED: OIL OF THE LEAVES

Tea tree oil was discovered in 1770 by Captain James Cook and botanist Sir John Banks while on an expedition to Australia. The aborigines were known to chew on the leaves, so

Banks collected samples of the leaves and took them to England for further studies. Tea tree oil has traditionally been used used as a medicinal agent for cuts, burns, bites and many skin ailments. Research done in the 1950s and early 1960s found the oil to be a germicide and fungicide with the additional characteristics of dissolving pus and debris. Recent studies have found it effective for the cure of thrush, vaginal infections, candida, staph infections, athlete's foot, hair and scalp problems, mouth sores, muscle and joint pain, pain, and boils. It has been found that tea tree oil is a very complex substance containing forty-eight different compounds. The compounds consist mainly of terpinenes, cymones, pinenes, terpineols, cinerol, sesquiterpenes, and sesquiterpene alcohols. All these work together in synergy to produce maximum healing power.

### PRIMARY APPLICATIONS

| | |
|---|---|
| Boils | Candida |
| Infections | Joint pain |
| Skin disorders | Staph and strep infections |

### SECONDARY APPLICATIONS

| | |
|---|---|
| Athlete's foot | Bruises |
| Burns | Fungus |
| Insect bites | Mouth sores |
| Muscle pain | Thrush |

# THYME (*Thymus vulgaris*)

### PARTS USED: ENTIRE PLANT

Thyme is a powerful antiseptic and general tonic with healing powers. It is used in cases of anemia and bronchial and intestinal disturbances. It is also used as an antiseptic against tooth decay. It destroys fungal infections such as athlete's foot and skin parasites like crabs and lice. Centuries ago, the herbalist Culpeper stated that thyme kills worms in the belly and that an ointment of thyme takes away any hot swelling and warts. This herb contains B-complex vitamins and vitamins C and D. It also contains iodine and some sodium, silicon and sulphur.

## PRIMARY APPLICATIONS

| | |
|---|---|
| Bronchitis, acute | Colic |
| Digestion | Gas |
| Gout, external | Headaches |
| Laryngitis | Lung congestion |
| Sciatica | Throat problems |

## SECONDARY APPLICATIONS

| | |
|---|---|
| Appetite stimulant | Asthma |
| Bowel problems | Bruises |
| Diarrhea | Epilepsy |
| Fainting | Fevers |
| Gastritis | Heartburn |
| Hysteria | Infection, internal |
| Mastitis | Menstruation, suppressed |
| Paralysis | Parasites |
| Perspiration (promotes) | Rheumatism |
| Sinus problems | Sprains |
| Stomach problems | Uterine problems |

# UVA URSI (*Arctostaphylos uva-ursi*)

PART USED: *LEAVES*

Uva ursi strengthens and tones the urinary passages and increases the flow of urine. It is especially beneficial for bladder and kidney infections. It is also useful for arthritis and cystitis. This herb is best known as the diabetes remedy for excessive sugar. Tincture of uva ursi was routinely prescribed in many European hospitals as a postpartum medicine to reduce hemorrhaging and help restore the womb to normal size. It should not be used during pregnancy in any large quantities because of the possibility of decreased circulation to the fetus.

## PRIMARY APPLICATIONS

Bladder infections          Bright's disease
Cystitis                    Diabetes
Gonorrhea                   Kidney infections
Nephritis                   Spleen
Urethritis, chronic         Uterine, ulceration

## SECONDARY APPLICATIONS

Arthritis                   Bedwetting
Bronchitis                  Diarrhea
Dysentery                   Female troubles
Gallstones                  Gravel
Hemorrhoids                 Liver
Lung congestion             Menstruation, excessive
Pancreas                    Prostate weakness

# VALERIAN *(Valeriana officinalis)*

### PART USED: ROOT

Valerian is a strong nervine. It contains an essential oil and alkaloids which combine to produce a calming sedative effect. Valerian is known as a safe non-narcotic herbal sedative and has been recommended for people who suffer from anxiety and/or insomnia. It is commonly used with other herbs for nervous tension. It is also useful in pain-relieving remedies and for its ability to relax muscle spasms. Valerian is rich in magnesium, potassium, copper, some lead and zinc. This herb is usually recommended for short-term use. Prolonged or excessive use can cause mental depression in some people. It is usually not recommended for small children.

## PRIMARY APPLICATIONS

| | |
|---|---|
| Convulsions | High blood pressure |
| Hysteria | Hypochondria |
| Nervousness | Pain |

## SECONDARY APPLICATIONS

| | |
|---|---|
| Alcoholism | Bronchial spasms |
| Colds | Coughs |
| Despondency | Drug addiction |
| Epilepsy | Gravel bladder |
| Head, congestion | Insomnia |
| Measles | Menstruation (promotes) |
| Muscle pain | Palpitations |
| Palsy | Scarlet fever |
| Shock | Spasms |
| Ulcers | Worms (expels) |

# VIOLET *(Viola odorata)*

## PARTS USED: FLOWERS AND LEAVES

Violet is very effective in healing internal ulcers. It is also used internally and externally for tumors, boils, abscesses, pimples, swollen glands and malignant growths. The properties in violet leaves and flowers seem to have abilities to reach places that only the blood and lymphatic fluids penetrate. It is useful to eliminate symptoms of difficult breathing caused by gas, distention and pressure. Violet contains vitamins A and C.

## PRIMARY APPLICATIONS

| | |
|---|---|
| Asthma | Bronchitis |
| Cancer | Colds, head congestion |
| Coughs | Sinus catarrh |
| Tumors | Ulcers |

## SECONDARY APPLICATIONS

| | |
|---|---|
| Breathing, difficult | Gout |
| Headaches | Sores |
| Syphilis | Throat, sore |

# WATERCRESS (*Nasturtium officinale*)

## PARTS USED: ENTIRE PLANT

Watercress is used principally as a tonic for regulating metabolism and the flow of bile. It helps in increasing physical endurance and stamina. Eaten fresh daily watercress is a very useful blood purifier and tonic to help supply needed vitamins and minerals. The juice of the leaves can be applied to the face for freckles, pimples, spots. It should be left overnight then washed off in the morning. Watercress soaked in honey has been found beneficial as a cough medicine. This herb is an excel-lent food for enriching the blood and a good remedy for most blood and skin disorders. Experiments have proven that the dried leaves contain three times as much vitamin C as the leaves of lettuce. Watercress is very rich in vitamins A, C, and D. It is one of the best sources of vitamin E. It also contains vitamins B and G and is high in iron, iodine, calcium, copper, sulphur and manganese.

## PRIMARY APPLICATIONS

| | |
|---|---|
| Anemia | Cramps |
| Kidney problems | Liver problems |
| Nervous ailments | Rheumatism |

SECONDARY APPLICATIONS

| | |
|---|---|
| Acne | Appetite (increases) |
| Cysts | Eczema |
| Heart (strengthens) | Joints, stiff |
| Kidney stones | Lactation |
| Mental disorders | Tuberculosis |
| Tumors, internal | Uterine cysts |

# WHITE OAK BARK (Quercus alba)

PART USED: BARK

White oak bark contains strong astringent properties that can be used for both external and internal bleeding. It is an excellent cleanser for skin and mucous membranes and heals damaged tissues in the stomach and intestines. It has been used for excess stomach mucus which causes the common complaint of sinus congestion and post-nasal drip. It also relieves the stomach by strengthening it for better internal secretion and absorption. In this way white oak bark indirectly influences metabolism. A tea made from the bark can be used with success as a wash for gum infection, a gargle for sore throats, and as an intestinal tonic for diarrhea. It is also used as an antidote for drug allergies and chemotherapy side-effects. This herb is useful for inflammations, abrasions, and cuts since it has a clotting, shrinking and antiseptic effect. White oak bark contains vitamin B12, calcium, phosphorus, potassium and iodine. It also has sulphur, iron, sodium, cobalt, lead, strontium, and tin.

PRIMARY APPLICATIONS

| | |
|---|---|
| Bleeding, internal and external | Bloody urine |
| Menstrual problems | Mouth sores |
| Skin irritations | Teeth |
| Throat, strep | Ulcers |

## SECONDARY APPLICATIONS

Bites, insect and snake
Cancer, prostate
Diarrhea
Gangrene
Goiter
Hemorrhoids
Kidneys
Nausea
Spleen problems
Uterus
Varicose Veins
Vomiting

Bladder problems
Dental problems
Fever (reduces)
Glandular swellings
Gums, sore
Indigestion
Liver
Pyorrhea
Tonsillitis
Vagina
Venereal diseases
Worms, pin

# WHITE PINE BARK (*Pinus strobus*)

## PART USED: BARK

White pine bark has medicinal properties as well as food value. Native Americans used to soak the bark in water until it became soft, then applied it to wounds. They also boiled the inner bark of saplings and drank the liquid for dysentery. The bark is also said to be an excellent expectorant, and to reduce mucus secretions present with common colds. White pine bark is rich in vitamin C and has some vitamin A. It contains iodine, calcium, copper, sodium, nickel, zinc and manganese.

## PRIMARY APPLICATIONS

Bronchitis
Laryngitis

Dysentery
Mucus

## SECONDARY APPLICATIONS

Colds
Flu

Croup
Kidney problems

| | |
|---|---|
| Lung congestion | Rheumatism |
| Scurvy | Strep throat |
| Tonsillitis | Whooping cough |

# WILD CHERRY (*Prunus virginiana*)

PART USED: BARK

Wild cherry is considered a very useful expectorant and is a valuable remedy for all catarrhal conditions. It is beneficial for bronchial disorders caused by the hardened accumulation of mucus. Wild cherry also contains a volatile oil which acts as a local stimulant in the alimentary canal and aids in digestion. It is a useful tonic for those convalescing because it tones up the entire system.

## PRIMARY APPLICATIONS

| | |
|---|---|
| Asthma | Bronchitis |
| Catarrh | Coughs (loosens) |
| Fever | High blood pressure |
| Mucus, hardened | Phlegm (loosens) |

## SECONDARY APPLICATIONS

| | |
|---|---|
| Diarrhea | Stomach, irritated |
| Eye sight | Flu |
| Gallbladder | Heart palpitation |

# WILD LETTUCE (*Lactuca virosa*)

PARTS USED: ENTIRE PLANT

Wild lettuce has been used to increase urine flow and to soothe sore and chapped skin. Native Americans used it as a tea for lactation. The leaves contain sedative properties that act somewhat like morphine, only milder. It is the dried leaves which are used to induce sleep and treat severe nervous disorders. The juice of the plant has also been used to relieve poison ivy.

### PRIMARY APPLICATIONS

| | |
|---|---|
| Bronchitis | Cramps |
| Nervous disorders | Pain, chronic |

### SECONDARY APPLICATIONS

| | |
|---|---|
| Asthma | Colic |
| Coughs | Diarrhea |
| Dropsy | Insomnia |
| Lactation | Spasms |

# WILD YAM (*Dioscorea villosa*)

### PART USED: ROOT

Wild yam is useful in glandular balance formulas for treating nausea in pregnant women. It is said to be an excellent preventive of miscarriage and also useful for cramps in the region of the uterus during later stages of pregnancy. Wild yam is useful for pain with gallstones. It will relax muscular fibers and soothe the nerves.

### PRIMARY APPLICATIONS

| | |
|---|---|
| Arthritis | Asthma, spasmodic |
| Bowel spasms | Colic, bilious |
| Gas | Liver problems |
| Menstrual cramps | Nausea (from pregnancy) |

### SECONDARY APPLICATIONS

| | |
|---|---|
| Boils | Bronchitis |
| Catarrh, stomach | Cholera |

| | |
|---|---|
| Hiccups, spasmodic | Jaundice |
| Nervousness | Neuralgia |
| Rheumatism | Scabies |

# WILLOW *(Salix)*

*PART USED: BARK*

Willow is valued as a nerve sedative because it has no depressing after-effects. It works like aspirin except that it is mild on the stomach. Traditionally, a bitter drink was made by steeping willow bark and twigs in water. This drink was used for fever and chills, and as a substitute for chinchona bark. Willow bark extract is helpful in cleansing and healing eyes that are inflamed or infected. It has been called one of the essential first aid plants. It has strong but benign antiseptic abilities and is good for infected wounds, ulcerations, or eczema.

## PRIMARY APPLICATIONS

| | |
|---|---|
| Eczema | Fever |
| Headache | Nervousness |
| Pain | Rheumatism |
| Sex depressant | Ulceration |

## SECONDARY APPLICATIONS

| | |
|---|---|
| Bleeding | Chills |
| Corns | Dandruff |
| Diarrhea | Dysentery |
| Earache | Flu |
| Gout | Hayfever |
| Heartburn | Impotence |
| Infection | Inflammation |
| Muscle, sore | Night sweats |
| Ovarian pain | Tonsillitis |

# WINTERGREEN *(Gaultheria procumbens)*

*PARTS USED:* LEAVES, OIL

Wintergreen is very valuable when used in small doses. It stimulates the stomach, heart and respiration. It has a penetrating effect on every cell and acts on the cause of pain. As a tea or hot compress it is beneficial for headaches, rheumatic pains, sciatica, and pains in the joints or muscles. An infusion may also be used as a gargle for sore throat or as a douche for leucorrhea. Externally, the oil of wintergreen has been used for rheumatism, warts, corns, callouses, cysts, and even tatoo marks.

## PRIMARY APPLICATIONS

| | |
|---|---|
| Aches and pains | Headaches, migraine |
| Gout | Lumbago |

## SECONDARY APPLICATIONS

| | |
|---|---|
| Cystitis | Diabetes |
| Diphtheria | Gas |
| Inflammation | Leucorrhea |
| Rheumatic fever | Sciatica |
| Throat gargle | Urinary |
| Yeast infections | |

# WITCH HAZEL *(Hamamelis virginiana)*

*PART USED:* BARK

Witch hazel is used externally as an alcohol extract for insect bites, varicose veins, burns, hemorrhoids and to stop bleeding wounds. It is used internally to help stop bleeding from the lungs, uterus and other internal organs. It is used as a mouth wash for bleeding gums and inflamed conditions of the mouth and throat. It is safe to use because of its mild and gentle action. Witch hazel contains vitamins C, E, K, and P. It also contains iodine, manganese, zinc, copper and selenium.

### PRIMARY APPLICATIONS

| | |
|---|---|
| Bleeding, internal | Gums |
| Hemorrhoids | Mucous membranes |
| Varicose veins | |

### SECONDARY APPLICATIONS

| | |
|---|---|
| Bruises | Burns |
| Cuts | Diarrhea |
| Dysentery | Eyes (bags) |
| Hemorrhage | Insect bites |
| Menstruation, excess | Muscles, sore |
| Scalds | Sinus |
| Swelling | Tuberculosis |
| Tumors | Venereal disease |

# WOOD BETONY (*Betonica officinalis*)

*PARTS USED: ENTIRE PLANT*

Wood betony is an effective sedative for children and a good tranquilizer for adults. It is useful for head and facial pain. It works in cleansing impurities from the blood and opens congested areas of the liver and spleen. It is said to be effective for many diseases. Wood betony contains magnesium, manganese and phosphorus.

### PRIMARY APPLICATIONS

| | |
|---|---|
| Delirium | Fevers |
| Headaches, migraine | Jaundice |
| Liver problems | Nervousness |

## Secondary Applications

Asthma, bronchial
Bleeding, internal
Convulsions
Epilepsy
Gout
Heart stimulant
Insanity
Lung congestion
Night sweats
Perspiration
Varicose veins

Bladder
Blood, improves
Diarrhea
Fainting
Heartburn
Indigestion
Kidney
Neuralgia
Pain
Stomach cramps

# WORMWOOD (*Artemisia absinthium*)

## Parts Used: *plant and leaves*

Wormwood is useful for complaints of the digestive system, such as constipation and indigestion. It is useful to stimulate sweating in dry fevers and for stomach acidity. It also has a stimulating effect on uterine circulation, promotes menstruation and will help relieve discomfort caused by cramps. It has been used externally and internally to check falling of hair and baldness. Wormwood contains vitamins C and B-complex. It also has manganese, calcium, potassium, sodium and small amounts of cobalt and tin. Wormwood is best used in small quantities and for short periods of time. It is rarely given to children.

## Primary Applications

Constipation
Debility
Fever
Labor pains (relieves)
Stomach problems

Cramps, menstrual
Digestion aids
Jaundice
Liver problems

## SECONDARY APPLICATIONS

| | |
|---|---|
| Appetite, increase | Blood circulation |
| Dropsy | Earaches |
| Female problems | Gallbladder |
| Gout | Insect (repels) |
| Kidney problems | Menstruation (promotes) |
| Morning sickness | Nausea |
| Obesity | Poisons (expels) |
| Rheumatism | Tonic |

# YARROW *(Achillea millefolium)*

*PART USED: FLOWER*

Yarrow is used as a tonic in helping to regulate the function of the liver. It tones mucous membranes of the stomach and bowels, and heals the glandular system. It also acts as a blood cleanser and at the same time opens pores to permit free perspiration, elimination of waste and relief of the kidneys. Yarrow leaves stimulate clotting in cuts and abrasions. This herb is valuable because it has a wide range of uses. It is even being studied as a possible anticancer agent. Yarrow contains vitamins A, C, E, and F and some vitamin K. It contains manganese, copper, potassium, iodine and iron.

## PRIMARY APPLICATIONS

| | |
|---|---|
| Blood cleanser | Bowels, hemorrhage |
| Catarrh | Colds |
| Fevers | Flu |
| Lungs, hemorrhage | Measles |
| Nosebleeds | Perspiration, obstructed |

## SECONDARY APPLICATIONS

| | |
|---|---|
| Abrasions | Ague |
| Appetite (stimulates) | Bladder |
| Brights disease | Bronchitis |
| Bruises | Burns |
| Cancer | Chicken pox |
| Cramps | Cuts |
| Diarrhea (infants) | Epilepsy |
| Hair, falling out | Headaches |
| Hysteria | Jaundice |
| Menstrual bleeding | Nipples, sore |
| Pneumonia | Rheumatism |
| Stomach problems | Sweating (promotes) |
| Ulcers | Urine retention |

# YELLOW DOCK (Rumex crispus)

## PART USED: ROOT

Yellow dock is an astringent and blood purifier so is useful in treating diseases of the blood and chronic skin ailments. It is one of the best blood builders in the herb kingdom. It stimulates elimination and improves bile flow. It is a nutritive tonic high in iron and very useful in treating anemia. This herb nourishes the spleen and liver and is therefore effective in treating jaundice, lymphatic problems, and skin eruptions. A high amount of easily digestible iron is found in yarrow. It is also rich in vitamins A and C, manganese and nickel.

## PRIMARY APPLICATIONS

| | |
|---|---|
| Anemia | Blood purifier |
| Itching | Eyelids, ulcerated |
| Liver congestion | Rheumatism |
| Skin problems | |

## SECONDARY APPLICATIONS

| | |
|---|---|
| Bladder | Blood disorders |
| Bowels, bleeding | Bronchitis, chronic |
| Cancer | Constipation |
| Dyspepsia | Ears, running |
| Female weakness | Jaundice |
| Leprosy | Leukemia |
| Lungs, bleeding | Lymphatic problems |
| Scurvy | Spleen |
| Stomach problems | Thyroid glands |
| Tumors | Ulcers |

# YERBA SANTA

*(Eriodictyon californicum, Benth.)*
PART USED: *LEAVES*

Yerba santa is a mild but useful decongestant. It is used for all forms of bronchial congestion and is an excellent remedy for chest conditions, acute and chronic. It is an herb that purifies the blood and stimulates all digestive secretions. The fresh or dried leaves of this herb were traditionally used by Native Americans as a poultice for both broken and unbroken skin. It is also used for pain resulting from rheumatism, tired limbs, swellings and sores.

## PRIMARY APPLICATIONS

| | |
|---|---|
| Asthma | Bronchial congestion |
| Colds | Hay fever |

## SECONDARY APPLICATIONS

| | |
|---|---|
| Bladder catarrh | Coughs |
| Diarrhea | Dysentery |
| Fever | Flu |
| Hemorrhoids | Kidney problems |

Laryngitis, chronic
Rheumatism
Throat, sore

Nose discharge
Stomach aches
Vomiting

# YOHIMBE (Pausinystalia johimbe)

PART USED: BARK

Yohimbe is a tree is found growing throughout Africa. It has gained popularity because of its use as an aphrodisiac. Compounds found in yohimbe are known to be precursors of testosterone, and the herb is thought to help with both female and male sexual dysfunction and impotency. Yohimbe dilates blood vessels near the skin, mucous membranes, and sex organs. This may cause fatigue in individuals with low blood pressure. Yohimbe should also be avoided by those with blood pressure or heart irregularities.

## PRIMARY APPLICATIONS

Impotency
Aphrodisiac

Sexual dysfunction

# YUCCA (Yucca glauca)

PART USED: ROOT

Yucca was used by the Indians of the Southwest for skin disorders, eruptions, and slow-healing ulcerations. It was also used on cuts to stop bleeding and help avoid inflammation. Native Americans also used the root as a poultice on breaks and sprains and for rheumatism. The properties of yucca which help in arthritis and rheumatism are due to the plant's high content of steroid saponins, which are precursors to cortisone. Some researchers feel that yucca saponins improve the body's ability to produce its own cortisone by supplying materials needed for the hormone to be manufactured by the adrenal glands. Yucca root is rich in vitamins A, B-complex, and has some vitamin C. It is high in calcium, potassium, phosphorus, iron, manganese and copper.

## PRIMARY APPLICATIONS

Arthritis                                 Rheumatism

## SECONDARY APPLICATIONS

Addison's disease             Blood purifier
Bursitis                               Cholesterol, reduces
Dandruff                           Gallbladder
Gonorrhea                         Inflammation, internal
Liver problems                  Skin irritations
Skin problems                   Venereal disease

# SECTION 3

# *Beyond Herbs— The Value of Supplements*

# Nutritional Supplements

## BLUE-GREEN ALGAE
*(Chloroplast membrane sulfolipids)*

**B**lue green algae is well known for its great nutritional value. Scientists at the National Cancer Institute have reported that blue-green algae may help protect against the AIDS virus. It has been found that algae helps the body produce interferon, a key component of the immune system. Because it can help strengthen the immune system, it is useful for growing children.

Blue-green algae is rich in nutrients that help balance the body chemistry and build resistance to viral diseases. It is known to increase the oxygen utilized by the body and is excellent to use in cases of acute diseases such as colds, flu, and fevers. It is rich in essential amino acids such as isoleucine, leucine, lysine, methionine, cystine, phenylalanine, tyrosine, and tryptophan. These amino acids are the raw materials of which the DNA is constructed. They provide material for bones, tissue, organs, hormones, neurotransmitters, enzymes, and they work to support the immune system. Blue-green algae is high in beta-carotene which is stored in the liver and used by the body as needed. It protects the lungs against air pollution. Blue-green algae is high in vitamin C, an antioxidant which is needed on a daily basis by the body. Algae also contains thiamin, riboflavin, and niacin, components of the B-complex vitamins. Beyond that it contains choline, biotin, pantothenic acid, vitamin K, iodine, calcium, phosphorus, magnesium, potassium, copper, iron, manganese, zinc, and sodium.

# MELATONIN

Melatonin is a hormone found naturally in the body. It is secreted by the pineal gland and contributes to the setting of the body clock. As daylight disappears, the eyes send a signal to the brain which in turn signals the pineal gland to start pumping melatonin. This causes a drop in body temperature, a slowing of the body's metabolism and sleepiness. When sunlight appears, the pineal gland turns off and the body awakens. This process continues through life, but the secretion of melatonin seems to decrease with age. This may be one contributing factor for increased sleeping problems that occur with age.

Melatonin has helped many individuals with sleep disorders. Even pharmaceutical companies are rushing to get in on the action by preparing prescription medications using melatonin. Melatonin can help promote sleep and relieve insomnia and restlessness. Some people who travel frequently have used melatonin to ease jet lag problems. When traveling, melatonin can be taken allow the body to adjust to a new sleep cycle. Some recommend one milligram of melatonin for each hour of time change.

Evidence shows that melatonin has even more benefits than good sleep. Research points to its powerful antioxidant properties. It may help improve the immune response and its anti-aging capabilities are also being explored. Some preliminary animal studies point to improvements in health and longer life span. Life was prolonged by about 25 percent in mice treated with melatonin. Evidence is mounting as to the benefits of melatonin for many serious ailments and problems. It may be too soon to know for sure, but melatonin seems to be a promising supplement for many conditions.

# DHEA *(Dehydroepiandrosterone)*

*D*HEA has garnered a lot of interest in the past several years. Numerous articles have published amazing information on this essential hormone. Claims have been made concerning its ability to slow the aging process, prevent cancer, aid diabetes, increase immune response and fight many different diseases. Generally it is thought that normal amounts of DHEA are beneficial for the body while lower amounts may lead to disease.

DHEA is a naturally occurring hormone made in the adrenal glands. It is the most abundant hormone found in the body and is sometimes referred to as the "mother hormone." It is a precursor hormone that can be metabolized into other adrenal hormones and acts with other hormones. When hormone levels are too low or out of sync, the body fails to function properly. Levels of DHEA in the body reach their peak at around 21 years of age and then tend to decline over the years.

Normal levels of DHEA can help to balance the immune system in fighting disease and infection. This protects the body from may serious problems that can occur such as cancer. The full extent of the benefits of DHEA are not entirely known. But there is evidence that links low levels of DHEA to conditions such as cancer, Alzheimer's disease, arthritis, osteoporosis, chronic fatigue syndrome, diabetes, fertility problems, lupus, rheumatoid arthritis, multiple sclerosis, allergies, PMS, and even weight problems. DHEA is being looked on by some as the single most important factor in maintaining health.

DHEA therapy has been shown to be free of side effects when taken in proper amounts. Some problems with excess amounts in the form of supplements include acne, rapid heart beat, irritability and headaches. Most have solved the problem by lowering the amount being taken.

It is impressive that a hormone found commonly in the body could offer such advantages to health. And even more important are the debilitating conditions that can result when there is too little DHEA available. It is produced in the adrenal glands and helps with manufacturing many other hormones form the adrenal glands. Adequate levels are essential to life.

# COENZYME Q-10

Coenzyme Q-10 (Co Q-10), also known as ubiquinone, is one of the most important nutrients known to man. There are ten different coenzymes, but only Co Q-10 is found in human tissue, in every cell of the body. This enzyme is an essential nutrient, an important antioxidant, and aids in the activity of other enzymes. Co Q-10 can be synthesized in the body, but deficiencies are fairly common as the ability of the body to synthesize the enzyme decreases with age.

Co Q-10 is a primary ingredient of cellular mitochondria. It is a catalyst in the production of energy and boosts biochemical ability. It is found in high concentrations in organs that require abundant amounts of energy such as the heart and liver. Co Q-10 is similar to vitamins E and K in its chemical structure. It is also thought to resemble vitamin E in its ability to function as an antioxidant. It has the ability to neutralize free radicals which cause damage to the cells. Because of the immune enhancing abilities of this enzyme, it may help with conditions such as AIDS, cancer, viral and bacterial infections, and tumors.

Co Q-10 has shown significant benefits when used by cardiac patients. The heart muscle needs this essential nutrient to function properly. When there is a deficiency, a myriad of cardiovascular problems can occur. Clinical tests have shown favorable results with heart patients taking Co Q-10. The coenzyme may help protect the heart from damage suffered during a heart attack. It may also help reduce tissue damage which occurs during open heart surgery and may aid with heart transplant patients. Some researchers believe that just the addition of Co Q-10 to the diet will improve heart performance, even without exercise. One study confirmed this theory. Volunteers were given a daily dose of the enzyme for eight weeks. Oxygen utilization and exercise capacity of the heart both improved.

Co Q-10 is present in many foods such as wheat bran, beef heart, spinach, peanuts and rice and is also thought to be safe when taken as a supplement. Even high doses have not shown to cause serious side effects. Some minor cases of gastrointestinal problems have been reported, but complications are rare and not severe.

# ENZYMES

*E*nzymes are the protein-like substances formed in plants and animals. They are considered an essential component in all body functions, digestion and tissue repair. They act as catalysts in chemical reactions and speed up the processes in the body. They are important for sustaining life.

The body can manufacture enzymes, and they can also be attained in some foods. (Sprouts are the highest source of enzymes.) There are four main categories of food enzymes. These include 1) lipase, which serves to break down fat; 2) protease, which breaks down protein; 3) cellulase, which assists in breaking down cellulose; and 4) amylase, which breaks down starch. It is raw foods that contain enzymes. When food is cooked, the enzymes are depleted or entirely destroyed.

Enzymes are the only nutrients able to give the body energy necessary to function. There are around 700 different enzymes in the body which each perform a different function. If adequate amounts of the enzymes are not available, diseases may occur. Glands and organs in the body depend on the activity of the enzymes to function properly. Enzymes are needed during the digestion process; enzymes work with other nutrients to construct muscle tissue, bone, skin, and nerve cells; enzymes help with elimination by aiding to release toxins through the colon, kidneys, skin and lungs. When valuable enzymes are missing, the glands must try and manufacture them. This results in overwork and exhaustion.

# MORINDA CITRIFOLIA (NONI)

Morinda citrifolia, also known as noni, is a plant that grows in the South Pacific. The berries have long been known to help cure various diseases. One of noni's recognized powers is the ability to ease joint pain present in arthritic diseases. Arthritic pain may be caused in part by the body's inability to properly or completely digest proteins. These unused proteins form crystal-like deposits in the joints of the body. Noni helps to enhance protein digestion through enzymatic function, and thus may help to eliminate the occurrence of pain caused by protein deposits.

The alkaloid compounds found in morinda have proven themselves to effectively control or kill over six types of infectious bacterial strains including *Escherichia coli, Salmonella typhi, Shigella paradysenteriae,* and *Staphyloccus aureaus.* In addition, damnacanthal, a chemical compound found in noni, was able to inhibit the early antigen stage of the Epstein-Barr virus, a virus involved in diseases such as chronic fatigue syndrome.

Morinda citrifolia is known as a nutritive booster, antioxidant, pain killer, skin healing agent, and can be used for diabetes and drug addiction. It is excellent for the digestive system, endocrine system, urinary tract and cardiovascular system.

# NOPAL

Nopal is a cactus plant known as prickly pear. In the desert regions of Mexico it is often used as a food. Nopal is excellent for the digestive system because it contains pectin, mucilage and gums. It helps prevent fat, excessive starch and sugars from entering the bloodstream and adhering to the artery walls. It also acts as a natural diuretic, neutralizes toxins, cleans the lymphatic system, and lowers blood sugar in type II diabetes.

# Nopal

Nopal is a cactus plant in... and generally grow in the desert. Nto... prickly pear, is often referred to as Lord... Nopal is excellent for the digestive system, it cause hypertension, preventing... much as old gum... it held Pectin the... Excessive starch and sugar from entering the bloodstream and adhering to the artery walls. It also acts as a natural diuretic, neutralizes toxins, cleans the lymphatic system, and lowers blood sugar in type II diabetes.

# SECTION 4

# Good Herbs,
# Good Food,
# Good Health

# Ailments and Herbal Combinations

Humans have always been afflicted with a plethora of diseases and disorders. In our quest to cure ourselves of disease, we've discovered and developed many natural and synthetic drugs, supplements and therapies. This section outlines many common ailments (in alphabetical order), along with herbal combinations that are used to combat the specific disorders. Also listed are other uses of the combinations, along with nutritional supplements helpful for treating the disease, and the orthodox therapies used by conventional doctors.

One may ask why there is a need to combine herbs. The answer is that an herbal combination, because it consists of two or more herbs, can provide therapeutic benefits for a wider range of ailments in a safe and effective manner. Combined herbs can also condition reflexes in the body which will produce effects comparable to those of specific drugs without being as drastic or producing undesired side effects. Eventually, because of the combination's natural fortification of the immune and other systems, the body then can become more healthy and able to maintain health on its own. The focus of this section is on the various ailments and the herbal combinations.

# ALLERGIES

An allergy is an over-reaction of the body cells to foreign cells. An allergic person may be sensitive to only one allergen, but multiple sensitivities are the rule. The offending allergens could be inhalants, foods, drugs, infectious agents, eye contacts, or any number of environmental or food items. The most common reaction symptoms include hay fever, asthma, hives, high blood pressure, and unusual fatigue. Some doctors feel that allergies are due to excessive accumulation of waste in the body caused by incorrect diet, which many times leads to body to overreact in its efforts to rid itself of offending toxins.

## HERBAL COMBINATION NO. 1

*Boneset:* contains antiseptic and antiviral properties and promotes sweating to help in colds and flu. Promotes the production of interferon.

*Fenugreek:* contains antiseptic properties, dissolves hardened mucus, and rids the lungs and bronchial tubes of mucus and phlegm.

*Horseradish:* has antibiotic properties and is a strong stimulant to clear lungs and nasal passages of infections.

*Mullein:* relieves pain, relaxes the body, controls coughs, cramps and spasms. Loosens mucus from respiratory and lymphatic systems.

*Fennel:* expels phlegm from the throat, eliminates toxins from the body and purifies the blood. Aids digestion. This formula can also be used in liquid extract form.

## HERBAL COMBINATION NO. 2

*Burdock:* works as a blood purifier and antibiotic, has antifungal, cleansing and healing properties

*Goldenseal:* antibiotic properties for infections, cleans system, reduces inflammation

*Parsley:* rich in minerals and vitamins, has a tonic effect on the body, increases resistance to infections

*Althea:* relaxes bronchial tubes, removes mucus from lungs, has soothing and healing properties

*Chinese Ephedra:* contains bronchiodilating properties, relieves congestion from allergies, colds, flu, bronchitis and asthma

*Capsicum:* disinfects and stimulates the system to help with congestion. Increases circulation and healing.

*Horehound:* natural expectorant, tonic, diuretic. Helps clean liver and balance gland secretions. Good for coughs

*Yerba Santa:* contains decongestant properties, purifies the blood, and stimulates digestive secretions

## HERBAL COMBINATION NO. 3

*Fenugreek:* eliminates mucus and soothes mucous membranes. Acts as a tonic to the stomach, lungs, and intestinal tract

*Thyme:* has strong antibiotic properties and acts as a tonic to the intestinal system

## OTHER USES

| | |
|---|---|
| Asthma | Bronchitis |
| Mucus buildup | Sinus |
| Colds | Infections |
| Hay fever | Upper respiratory |

## SPECIAL DIETARY AIDS

*Vitamin A and Zinc:* work together to help increase antibodies in the system

*Vitamin B-complex:* necessary for vitality, mental energy and nerves

*Vitamins B2 and B6:* vital in the formation of antibodies

*Vitamin C and Pantothenic Acid:* vital in the production of adrenal hormones which give the system an antiallergic effect

*Vitamin D:* helps the body absorb calcium

*Vitamin E:* protects the cells against allergies

*Calcium:* works with enzymes for utilization

*Minerals:* a balanced mineral tablet will help eliminate allergies

*Bee Pollen:* Many allergies such as asthma or hay fever have been caused by pollen entering the respiratory system. Bee Pollen can build immunity by acting as a barrier against the inhaled pollens. Start with small amounts.

*Magnesium, selenium and zinc:* vital for the immune system. Deficiency of magnesium is seen in allergic persons.

*Essential Fatty Acids:* necessary to inhibit inflammation. Flaxseed, borage, evening primrose and salmon are good oils.

*Millet:* an alkaline grain rich in calcium and magnesium

*Digestive Enzymes:* necessary to break up undigested protein and food in the bloodstream so the body can eliminate them. Use after meals to assure food is digested and assimilated properly. Use between meals to eliminate toxins from the blood.

*Hydrochloric Acid:* necessary to assure protein is being digested.

*Brewer's Yeast, Grape Juice and Wheat Germ:* Nutrients in this blend helps the body strengthen its cells and walls to stop the infecting microbes. Has been called a natural immunity.

*Brown Rice:* nonallergenic with a low fiber content, easy for the glands to absorb.

*Fruits:* Stone fruits (apricots, peaches, plums, nectarines) will create a natural antibiotic in the blood stream to help build resistance and clean the system to ease sensitivity to allergies.

*Garlic:* Eating fresh garlic is a natural way to help fight allergies such as colds and bronchial spasms.

*Honey (Raw):* has been effective in the treatment of 90 percent of all allergies. Raw honey contains all the pollen dust and mold that cause 90 percent of all allergies.

*Nuts:* high in protein, unsaturated fats, minerals and vitamins and life-giving enzymes to build the blood to strengthen against allergies

*Avoid:* wheat products, all canned food, dairy products, citrus fruits (unless tree ripened), all sugar and salt

## ORTHODOX PRESCRIBED MEDICATION

Prednisone has been prescribed for hay fever. It is a cortisone-like medicine. Intake of cortisone-type medications must be tapered off slowly to allow the body to increase its own production. Typical side effects of these types of drugs include:

| | |
|---|---|
| Cataracts | Depletion of calcium |
| Depression | Indigestion |
| Infections (susceptible) | Stomach pain |
| Stomach upset | Ulcers |
| Water retention | |

# ANEMIA

Anemia is a condition in which there is a reduction in the number of circulating red blood cells. Some symptoms associated with severe anemia are weakness, vertigo, headaches, roaring in the ears, spots before the eyes, irritability, psychotic behavior, and fatigue. Anemia often arises from recurrent infections and/or diseases involving the entire body. It could also be caused by the poor intake or absorption of nutrients, or by the loss of blood caused by menstruation or peptic ulcers.

## HERBAL COMBINATION NO. 1

*Red Beet:* cleanses and stimulates the liver and spleen.
*Yellow Dock:* high in natural iron, and blood builder.

*Red Raspberry:* rich in calcium and iron

*Chickweed:* rich in iron, copper, vitamin C, calcium and sodium. Contains antiseptic properties and strengthens the stomach and bowels.

*Burdock:* high in iron, valuable for the blood, clears the blood of harmful acids.

*Nettle:* rich in iron, nourishing to the blood, tones the entire system.

*Mullein:* very high in iron, soothing to the nerves, pain killer, and removes mucus from the system.

*Rose Hips:* rich in iron and calcium, high in minerals and vitamins, helps protect against infections

*Thyme:* has tonic and antiseptic properties, healing for anemia, bronchitis and intestinal problems

## OTHER USES

| | |
|---|---|
| Convulsions | Cramps |
| Energy | Fatigue |
| Kidneys | Multiple Sclerosis |
| Parkinson's Disease | Pituitary Gland |
| Senility | |

## SPECIAL DIETARY AIDS

*Blue-green Algae:* rich in iron, B12, and all nutrients to nourish the blood, also eliminates toxins.

*Essential Fatty Acids:* important for nourishing the body. These include flaxseed, borage, evening primrose oil, salmon oil.

*B-Complex Vitamins:* especially B6 and B12, help to manufacture red blood cells

*Vitamin C:* aids in the absorption and retention of iron

*Vitamin E:* necessary for healthy red blood cells

*PABA:* effective in formation of blood cells

*Copper:* vital to the blood (along with iron)

*Folic Acid:* assists in formation of blood cells, metabolism of proteins

*Iron:* enriches the blood, develops red blood cells

*Manganese:* works like iron in the function of red blood cells

*Protein:* nourishes the cells and assists in metabolism

*Apples:* strengthens the blood, rich in vitamins and minerals

*Apricots:* rich in iron and copper, very beneficial in anemia

*Bananas:* rich in potassium

*Chicken Breast:* complete protein

*Green Drink:* rich in chlorophyll which is similar to human blood

*Dried Beans and Peas:* high in protein

*Egg Yolks:* high in protein

*Fresh, Raw Blackberries:* good blood cleanser and good for anemia

*Grains, Whole:* barley, millet, buckwheat and cornmeal contain natural protein and vitamin B-complex, create bulk in the bowels, nourish the blood and cells

*Raw Nuts and Seeds:* sunflower seeds, sesame seeds, raw almonds, cashews, rich in protein, vitamins, minerals, unsaturated fats and enzymes to build the blood

*Vegetables (Dark, Green, Leafy):* especially mustard greens, kale, swiss chard, beet greens, spinach, and collards, rich in enzymes and chlorophyll

*Vegetables, Yellow:* rich in enzymes and work as natural cleansers

## ORTHODOX PRESCRIBED MEDICATION

A combination of iron and liver injections is recommended for iron deficiency anemia and in certain nutritional deficiencies. Antacids given with iron compound will decrease the absorption or iron. Its side effects include:

| | |
|---|---|
| Constipation | Diarrhea |
| Gastrointestinal irritation | Nausea |

# ARTHRITIS

A rthritis is defined as inflammation and soreness of the joints, usually accompanied by pain and, frequently, changes in structure. The two main types are osteoarthritis and rheumatoid arthritis. Osteoarthritis develops as a result of the constant wearing away of the cartilage in a joint. Symptoms of osteoarthritis are body stiffness and pain in the joints during damp weather, in the morning, or after heavy exercise.

Rheumatoid arthritis affects the whole body, instead of just a joint. Emotional stress usually brings on the onset of the disease. Rheumatoid arthritis destroys the cartilage and tissues in and around the joints and sometimes on the bone surface. Symptoms include swelling and pain in the joints, fatigue, anemia, weight loss and fever.

## HERBAL COMBINATION NO. 1

*Bromelain:* helps in tension pain, reduces inflammation and swelling

*Yucca:* cleansing agent, precursor to synthetic cortisone

*Alfalfa:* contains alkaloid for pain and nutrients for body strength

*Black Cohosh:* relieves pain and irritation and acid

*Yarrow:* acts as a blood cleanser and is soothing to the mucous membranes, helps regulate function of the liver

*Capsicum:* stimulant, equalizes circulation, catalyst for other herbs

*Chaparral:* dissolves uric acid accumulations and acts as an antiseptic

*Burdock:* reduces swelling and deposits within joints and knuckles

*Hydrangea:* acts like cortisone with cleansing power, helps prevent deposits in joints, rich in minerals to help build joints.

*Horsetail:* rich in silica necessary for strong bones and cartilage, replaces needed minerals.

*Catnip:* contains relaxing properties which are necessary for the body to heal, also rich in vitamins and minerals.

*Valerian:* a safe herbal sedative, useful in pain-relieving formulas, rich in magnesium, potassium, copper and zinc.

*White Willow:* natural sedative to relieve pain, contains cleansing properties.

*Slippery Elm:* helps rebuild tissues and glands, eliminates toxins, heals joints and helps in the digestion of nutrients.

*Sarsaparilla:* increases circulation to joints, balances hormones, rich in minerals for healthy joints and bones.

## OTHER USES

| | |
|---|---|
| Blood cleanser | Bursitis |
| Calcification | Gout |
| Neuritis | Rheumatism |

## SPECIAL DIETARY AIDS

*Glucosamine Sulfate:* natural and safe to use, improves symptoms, boosts tissue regeneration. A true chondoprotective agent (cartilage). Absorbs easily and is nontoxic.

*Herbal Calcium Formula:* necessary to nourish the bones and joints; the formula consists of alfalfa, marshmallow, plantain, horsetail, oatstraw, wheat grass and hops.

*Cat's Claw:* Contains anti-inflammatory properties to eliminate inflammation and pain in the joints. A powerful immune system booster.

*Digestive Enzymes:* very essential to assure proper digestion and assimilation of nutrients. They will also help digest toxins and protein, viruses, and bacteria in the body so it can be eliminated.

*Essential Fatty Acids:* These include flaxseed, borage, black currant, evening primrose, and fish oils. Eliminate saturated fats from your diet and add EFAs. Improvement will be seen in arthritis. EFAs srengthen the glands and boost immune function.

*Vitamin A:* helps to combat infection

*Vitamin B:* helps in assimilating carbohydrates

*Vitamin C:* (rutin and bioflavonoid) strengthens the capillary walls in the joints from breaking down and causing pain, swelling and possibly bleeding. Need to take high amounts especially when taking aspirin.

*Histadine (natural amino acid):* has anti-inflammatory properties for rheumatoid arthritis. Avoid red meat which causes uric acid build-up.

*Bran:* two tablespoons in 8 oz. water daily helps keep colon clean

*Raw Fruits and Vegetables:* feed the glands and manufacture hormones

*Low Sodium Diet:* salt is toxic and causes retention of water in tissues

*Iron, B2, And Folic Acid:* useful in building the blood

*Green Drinks:* contain chlorophyll which, as an indirect action on bacteria, breaks down poisons

*Sprouts:* contains quality protein without uric acid build up. Full of enzymes, vitamins and minerals.

*Cod Liver Oil:* valued for vitamin D content. Lubricates the joints and cartilage

*Exercise:* useful to help prevent and treat arthritis because unused joints tend to stiffen

*Fast For Several Days:* introduce one food at a time to determine what foods may cause the pain of arthritis.

*Natural Fruit And Vegetables:* stay away from acid fruits, especially lemon

*Organic Honey And Brewer's Yeast:* the two natural hormone foods stimulate the adrenal glands, rejuvenating the joints, mobility of stiff fingers and limbs

*Protein From Whole Grains, Nuts And Seeds:* contains quality proteins, rich in vitamins, minerals and amino acids. Nuts and seeds do not result in the formation of excessive uric acid. Best with green vegetables, and must be chewed thoroughly.

*Taheebo Tea:* has helped many people eliminate arthritis. It cleans the blood and strengthens the body

*Whey Powder:* Rich in sodium, purifies the blood, prevents calcium from depositing in the walls of the arteries

## ORTHODOX PRESCRIBED MEDICATION

### ASPIRIN

Aspirin is commonly used in high doses (16 to 20 per day) to treat a wide variety of ills. Its common side effects include heartburn, nausea, ringing in the ears, stomach bleeding, stomach pain, stomach ulcers and vomiting.

### CORTISONE

Cortisone is a steroid-type medicine. It is prescribed to provide relief for inflamed areas of the body. Its common side effects include:

| | |
|---|---|
| Depletion of calcium | Depression |
| Electrolyte imbalance | Psychosis |
| Stomach ulcers | Susceptibility to infection |
| Water retention | |

# BLOOD PURIFIER

Impure blood is usually caused by poor action of the liver and bowels, faulty digestion or problems in the lymphatic glands which can be responsible for the accumulation of impurities in the blood. The number of toxins in the blood will vary with each person, as will the degree of resistance to disease. Toxins build up in the system to cause diseases. Toxemia is caused from eating too much of the wrong kinds of food, such as red meat, white sugar products, white flour products, coffee and cola drinks. Impurities in the air, food additives, and medicine of all kinds can also be a cause of impure blood.

## HERBAL COMBINATION NO. 1

*Pau d'Arco:* a blood cleanser with antibacterial properties, protects the liver, improves assimilation of nutrients and eliminates fungus infestations

*Buckthorn:* cleansing for the blood, liver and gallbladder. Calming and healing to the intestinal tract.

*Peach Bark:* healing properties, strengthens the nervous system, natural diuretic properties.

*Stillingia:* stimulates the liver and glandular system. It eliminates toxins from the blood.

*Prickly Ash:* a great stimulant to remove toxins from the blood and improve circulation.

*Yellow Dock:* nutritive tonic very high in iron, nourishes the liver and spleen

*Dandelion:* helps liver to detoxify poisons, blood purifier and cleanser, rich in vitamins and minerals

*Burdock:* blood purifier, promotes kidney function to clear the blood of harmful acids

*Red Clover:* eliminates toxins, full of valuable minerals and vitamins with high amounts of iron and vitamins

*Barberry:* promotes bile in liver to clean blood, removes morbid matter from stomach and bowels

*Cascara Sagrada:* safe laxative, stimulates the secretions of the digestive system

*Yarrow:* opens the pores and purifies the blood

*Sarsaparilla:* contains stimulating properties, noted for increasing the metabolic rate

## HERBAL COMBINATION NO. 2

*Red Clover:* cleans blood, dissolves deposits, natural diuretic, reduces inflammation, promotes tissue repair.

*Burdock:* excellent blood cleanser, prevents deposits from accumulating in joints, promotes hormone balance and is high in vitamin C and iron.

*Pau d'Arco:* natural antibiotic properties, protects liver, provides nutrients to assist the body in healing itself. Known to reduce tumors, helps in candida.

*Natural Spices:* enhance the benefits of all the herbs.

## HERBAL COMBINATION NO. 3

*Burdock:* great blood and lymphatic cleanser, balances hormones and prevents mineral deposits in joints.

*Sheep Sorrel:* blood purifier, cleans urinary tract, eliminates toxins, rich in calcium.

*Slippery Elm:* soothing and healing for the mucous membranes, neutralizes in the blood, nourishes while healing.

*Turkish Rhubarb:* cleans and nourishes the intestines and blood, neutralizes acids in the blood, good for liver problems

## OTHER USES

| | |
|---|---|
| Acne | Age spots |
| Anemia | Arthritis |
| Blood purifier | Boils |
| Cancer | Canker sores, cleansing |
| Colon | Constipation |
| Eczema | Erysipelas |
| Eruptions | Infections |
| Insect bites | Jaundice |
| Liver | Lymph glands |
| Pancreas | Poison ivy/oak |

Pruritus
Ringworm
Scurvy
Spleen
Tetters
Tumors
Uric acid buildup

Psoriasis
Rheumatism
Skin problems
Diabetes
Tonsillitis
Undulant fever
Venereal disease

## SPECIAL DIETARY AIDS

*Blue-green Algae, Chlorophyll, Spirulina:* rich in B12, calcium, clean and build the blood.

*Free-Form Amino Acids:* needed by the body for healing, protect the body from disease

*Essential Fatty Acids:* necessary for every function of the body

*Reishi Mushrooms:* cleans and protects the liver, has anti-inflammatory properties, kills viruses and bacteria, an antitumor agent, protects the immune system

*Shark Cartilage:* has anti-inflammatory properties and helps to control pain, used for cancer, psoriasis, and intestinal disorders

*Vitamin A:* promotes growth and repair of body tissues

*Vitamin B-complex:* important in stressful situations and healthy nerves

*Vitamin C And Rutin:* promotes healthy blood vessels

*Vitamin D:* improves absorption of calcium and phosphorus in the bloodstream

*Vitamin E:* dilates capillary blood vessels helping blood to flow more freely into muscle tissues

*Vitamin F:* improves heart action and increases circulation

*Kelp:* high in organic iron

*Lecithin And Niacin:* improve appetite, digestion, assimilation, and elimination

*Beet Greens:* high in iron and other minerals

*Chard:* rich in iron, helps purify the blood

*Cherries (sour):* a natural blood cleanser

*Garlic And Capsicum:* clean the blood of toxins

*Green Drink:* (made with alfalfa sprouts, spearmint, comfrey and parsley in unfiltered apple juice) cleans the blood

*Juices, Carrot And Celery:* contain vitamins and minerals to rejuvenate the system

*Lemons And Limes:* clean the system of impurities, neutralize excess acid, natural antiseptics

*Parsley:* rich in iron, cleans and builds the blood with its nutrients

*Spinach:* high in iron

*Strawberry:* helps remove metallic poisons from the blood

*Sprouts:* contain live enzymes to build the blood and purify the body

*Whole Grains (millet, buckwheat and barley):* contain essential protein and amino acids to withstand diseases

## Orthodox Prescribed Medication

### Cyclandelate (Vasodilators)

Cyclandelate increases the size of blood vessels and treats poor blood circulation. Its possible side effects include:

| | |
|---|---|
| Belching | Dizziness |
| Flushing of face | Headache |
| Heartburn | Nausea or stomach pain |
| Rapid heart beat | Sweating |

# BONE, FLESH AND CARTILAGE

The following herbs have been used successfully in healing bones. These herbs are combined to help nature heal wounds and repair bones. They are also useful in healing abrasions and burns. All the herbs in this combination contain zinc which has been found essential for rapid healing.

## HERBAL COMBINATION No. 1

*Comfrey:* heals wounds and bones, healing effect on whole system

*Goldenseal:* natural antibiotic with healing powers, stops infections, and contains healing vitamins and minerals

*Marshmallow:* rich in vitamin A, zinc, and calcium, aids in the formation of bones, flesh and cartilage, contains healing properties for lung ailments, reduces inflammation and infections, builds the immune system

*Plantain:* high in calcium and minerals for assimilation, clears the kidneys and lungs of mucus, reduces inflammation.

*Wheatgrass:* rich in calcium and minerals to enrich the blood and bones. High in chlorophyll for cleansing the blood and eliminating toxins.

*Hops:* calming for the nerves to speed healing, nourishes the liver and stomach restores appetite and reduces inflammation.

*Slippery Elm:* strengthens the body, nutritious, draws out impurities

*Aloe Vera:* natural detoxicants, removes morbid matter from body, heals and protects.

## OTHER USES

| | |
|---|---|
| Abrasions | Broken Bones |
| Burns | Cuts |
| Poultices | Wounds |

## SPECIAL DIETARY AIDS

*Vitamin A:* helps in skin wounds along with potassium

*Vitamin B Complex:* provides the body with energy, needed daily, water-soluble and does not store in body

*Vitamin C:* bioflavonoid, strengthens small blood vessels

*Vitamin D:* natural blood clotting agent, strengthens bones, necessary for calcium assimilation

*Vitamin E:* promotes and relieves healing

*Calcium:* essential in preventing breaks as well as a rapid healing process

*Dolomite:* bone meal, natural source of calcium, phosphorus, and magnesium

*Zinc:* necessary for strengthening tissues, speeds healing

*Broccoli:* contains calcium, high in vitamin A

*Grains:* especially sprouted, to lessen excess mucus, and are rich in calcium

*Green Vegetables:* high content of calcium

*Kale Leaves:* very high in calcium

*Milk Products:* high in calcium

*Parsley:* rich in calcium and other vital minerals

*Protein:* builds and repairs tissues

*Sauerkraut:* is rich in calcium, and is very healing and nourishing

*Seeds:* sesame, high in iron and very high in calcium

*Sprouts:* contains live enzymes quickly assimilated in the body

*Whey Powder:* high in sodium, dissolves any calcium deposits that might accumulate, the sodium in whey powder will help dissolve spurs on the spine

## ORTHODOX PRESCRIBED MEDICATION

Drugs have a definite effect on bone fractures. Patients who break bones and take dolomite found that their bones healed more rapidly. One excuse for doctors to justify prolonged use of estrogen is to prevent osteoporosis, a weakening of bones that comes with age. Corticosteroids do contribute to bones being brittle, but an intake of necessary calcium through the year would benefit.

# BONES, TEETH, AND CALCIUM DEFICIENCY

The bones serve as a storage place for mineral salts and play an important role in the formation of blood cells. They also give shape to and support the body. Calcium deficiency can cause tooth decay, muscle cramps, nervousness, restlessness, insomnia, loss of resistance against infections, poor circulation, bronchitis and colds, among other problems. High intake of meat can lead to mineral imbalance—too much phosphorus and too little calcium. This can lead to a calcium and magnesium deficiency and result in loss of teeth through decay and pyorrhea. Symptoms of calcium deficiency are brittle bones, poor development of bones and teeth, dental caries, rickets, tetany, extreme irritability, and excessive bleeding. Restlessness, insomnia, muscle cramps, back and leg pains, even asthma and hay fever are symptoms of calcium deficiency. Recently, a medical research has proposed that calcium deficiency is the major cause of high blood pressure.

## HERBAL COMBINATION NO. 1

*Comfrey:* high in calcium and phosphorus, blood cleanser, helps provide calcium and phosphorus for strong bones
*Horsetail:* rich in silica, which aids the circulation
*Oat Straw:* high in silicon, rich in calcium and phosphorus, helps prevent diseases
*Lobelia:* removes congestion within the blood vessels

## HERBAL COMBINATION NO. 2

*Comfrey:* feeds the pituitary to help strengthen the body skeleton, high in calcium and phosphorus

*Alfalfa:* high in easily assimilated vitamins and minerals, alkalizer for the whole system

*Oat Straw:* powerful stimulant, rich in body building materials, rich in calcium and silicon

*Irish Moss:* purifies and strengthens the cellular structure and vital fluids of the system, high in calcium

*Horsetail:* healing for fractured bones, rich in silica and selenium, strengthens the tissues

*Lobelia:* strengthens the muscular action of the vessel walls to promote health

## HERBAL COMBINATION NO. 3

*White Oak:* helps in reducing capillary fragility, high in B2, calcium, and minerals

*Comfrey:* strengthens skeleton, helps in calcium and phosphorus balance

*Mullein:* nourishes and strengthens the lungs, calms the nerves, aids in keeping the glands and lymphatic system in good condition, high in iron, magnesium, potassium and sulphur

*Black Walnut:* high in protein, contains silica, antiseptic, healing to the system

*Marshmallow:* rich in calcium, acts as a diuretic, tonic and soothing to the nerves

*Queen of the Meadow:* useful for all problems of joints, tonic, contains Vitamins A and D

*Wormwood:* helps in digestion of protein and fat, contains B-complex and vitamin C

*Lobelia:* healing powers with ability to remove congestion in blood vessels

*Skullcap:* strengthens the nerves, high in calcium, potassium and magnesium

## OTHER USES

| | |
|---|---|
| Aches | Allergies |
| Arteriosclerosis | Arthritis |
| Blood clotting | Bursitis |
| Cartilage | "Charlie Horses" |
| Colds | Colitis |
| Convulsions | Cramps |
| Female Problems | Flesh |
| Flu | Fractures |
| Growing Pains | Gout |
| Headaches | Heart Palpitations |
| High Blood Pressure | Hormonal Balance |
| Hypoglycemia | Infections |
| Insomnia | Joints |
| Lactation | Menstrual Cramps |
| Nerves | Pains |
| Pregnancy | Rheumatism |
| Teeth | Ulcers |
| Varicose Veins | Water Retention |
| Wounds | |

## SPECIAL DIETARY AIDS

*Vitamin A:* essential for healthy bones and teeth

*Vitamin B-complex:* assists body in absorption, feeds tissues

*Vitamin B12:* tones the muscles, acts as a nutrition stimulant

*Vitamin C:* assists healing of fractures, wounds and scar tissue

*Vitamin D:* essential for the absorption of calcium and phosphorus

*Vitamin E:* removes scar tissue, (external and internal)

*Bioflavonoid Complex:* works with vitamin C for healthy capillaries

*PABA:* function in metabolism of protein

*Calcium:* necessary in helping protein fibers to form a new bone

*Fluorine:* preserves bones

*Hydrochloric Acid:* helps in mineral assimilation

*Iodine:* necessary for development of physical growth
*Iron:* to build red blood cells
*Magnesium:* increases flexibility to bones and tissues
*Phosphorus:* assists maintenance of density in bone structure
*Protein:* necessary in proper healing
*Silica:* tones the entire system
*Zinc:* assists body in B-complex absorption, feeds tissues
*Almonds:* rich in calcium and protein
*Beans, Pinto:* contains calcium and protein
*Brewer's Yeast:* contains B vitamins and other essential nutrients
*Grains, Whole:* nourishing with proteins for building cells
*Greens, Collard, Kale Turnip, And Mustard:* high in calcium
*Kefir:* helps calcium to assimilate
*Kelp:* high in calcium
*Millet:* easily digested, high in protein
*Seeds, Sesame:* rich in calcium and protein

## ORTHODOX PRESCRIBED MEDICATION

### MILK

Milk intake is usually recommended. Because chocolate interferes with calcium absorption, chocolate milk can thereby limit calcium absorption. There has been research to show that too much meat leads to severe calcium deficiency.

Many older people lose their ability to digest milk and will develop gas, indigestion and diarrhea. (Lact-aid will help predigest milk sugar to eliminate this.) Though Tums are recommended as a source of calcium, you should understand they contain calcium carbonate, which is not the best source of calcium. Tums could even increase the risk of kidney stones and decrease the absorption of other essential minerals.

# BODY CLEANSING

*H*erbs can be very useful in a cleansing program. Cleansing diets are very important to help rid the body of harmful accumulations of toxins. Toxin accumulation is caused by eating the wrong foods, air pollution, drugs, or from diseases which cause putrefaction and decay in the stomach and intestines. These germs can cause a buildup of urinary waste in the bloodstream. These excess wastes that are not eliminated can turn to solid matter or slime. Many nutritionists recommend using herbs to empty the bowels before beginning a fast. Enemas can also be helpful. A buildup of toxic materials in the colon walls begin to decay and to form and build toxic materials which poison all areas of the body and give a general feeling of fatigue, nausea, depression, inability to do the necessary daily functions. A completely clean colon is necessary to help rid the body of diseases.

## Herbal Combination No. 1

*Gentian:* gives strength to the system, tones the stomach, cleans blood

*Irish Moss:* high in minerals, gives strength to system, soothes tissues of lungs and kidneys

*Goldenseal:* cleansing action on system, kills poisons, strengthens the body

*Fenugreek:* dissolves hardened mucus, kills infections, rich in vitamins and minerals

*Safflower:* clears cholesterol, eliminates gastric disorders, supports adrenal glands

*Myrrh:* heals colon and stomach, speeds healing action, stimulates blood flow

*Yellow Dock:* purifies blood, stimulates digestion, improves liver function

*Black Walnut:* burns up excess toxins in the system

*Barberry:* works on liver to help bile flow freely, removes morbid matter from stomach and bowels

*Dandelion:* gives nutrition to body, destroys acids in blood, eliminates toxins

*Chickweed:* helps curb appetite, dissolves plaque in blood vessels, strengthens stomach and bowels

*Catnip:* relieves fatigue, sedative to nerves, rids body of bacteria

*Cyani:* stimulating tonic for the body, antiseptic to the blood

*Parthenium:* contains blood and lymphatic cleansing properties similar to echinacea, natural diuretic, cleansing for the bladder and kidneys.

*Cascara Sagrada:* cleans and restores bowel function. Helps eliminate built-up glue-like material on the colon walls.

*Slippery Elm:* contains nourishing and healing properties. Soothes and heals while cleansing and restoring the intestinal tract.

*Uva Ursi:* heals and strengthens the urinary tract. It contains antiseptic properties to heal infections.

## OTHER USES

| | |
|---|---|
| Arthritis | Cancer |
| Colon | Constipation |
| Pain | Parasites |
| Skin Problems | Toxic Wastes |
| Tumors | Worms |

## SPECIAL DIETARY AIDS

*Vitamin A:* helps repair body tissues

*Vitamin C:* detoxifies and promotes healthy blood vessels

*Vitamin D:* helps maintain healthy bones and teeth

*Vitamin E:* reduces uric acid, dilates capillary blood vessels helping blood flow more freely

*Mineral Supplements:* vital to mental and physical well-being

*Acidophilus:* keeps intestines clean

*Calcium:* helps build blood

*Lecithin:* helps maintain cell health, reduces cholesterol level in the blood

*Green Drinks:* clean the body, contain chlorophyll

*Juices, Unfiltered Apple Juice, Cranberry, And Grape:* nourish and clean the body

*Lemon Peel:* contains rutin to strengthen the capillaries

*Papaya:* cleans the intestines

*Teas, Herbal:* Red Raspberry, Mints, Taheebo, clean the system

*Vegetable Broths:* to strengthen the body, high in potassium

*Water, Pure:* cleans the system

## ORTHODOX PRESCRIBED MEDICATION

### MALTSUPEX

This often-prescribed medication is a bulk-forming laxative. Its common side effects:

| | |
|---|---|
| Nerve damage | Muscle damage |
| Chronic digestive disorder | |

# COLDS, FLUS AND FEVERS

Colds are very contagious. The common cold brings about inflammation of the mucous membranes of the respiratory pas sages caused by viruses. It is the body's way of trying to get rid of toxins and poisons built up in the body. An acute catarrhal infection, chills, scratchy throat, sneezing, aches in the back, cough, stuffy nose, and headache. Several herbs are known to help relieve the symptoms of the flu and cold, and many help to strengthen the immune system, which, in turn, helps rid the body completely of the condition. For instance, fenugreek and thyme help decongest the sinuses and garlic is a powerful antibiotic. Refer to the following combinations for more information on herbs and their uses for the cold and flu.

## HERBAL COMBINATION NO. 1.

*Rose Hips:* rich in vitamin C (well-known for fighting colds), helps inflamed ears, eyes, nose and throat.

*Chamomile:* works on inflammations in ear, eyes, nose and throat and acts as a sedative

*Slippery Elm:* removes mucus from system, soothing to lungs in colds and coughs

*Yarrow:* purifies the blood of waste material, effective for fevers

*Capsicum:* stimulant to warm the system, helps lower fevers and increases the power of other herbs

*Goldenseal:* natural antibiotic, helps stop infection and heals mucous membranes

*Myrrh Gum:* contains antiseptic properties, used as a tonic to stimulate lungs and bronchials

*Peppermint:* excellent for nausea, good for chills, cleans and strengthens the system

*Sage:* good for excessive mucus discharge, good for fever and lungs

*Lemon Grass:* used as an antifever herb for flu, colds and fevers, high in Vitamin A

## HERBAL COMBINATION NO. 2

*Boneset:* excellent for flu and colds, stimulates the liver, and eliminates toxins, strengthens the stomach and spleen.

*Fenugreek:* dissolves and softens built-up mucous in the body, antiseptic properties, dissolves cholesterol, soothes and nourishes during colds, flu and fevers.

*Horseradish:* antibiotic properties, strong stimulant properties to clear nasal passages and clear infections. Rich in vitamin C, sulphur and potassium which help to heal from colds, flu and fevers.

*Mullein:* relieves pain and relaxes the body, loosens mucus to be eliminated by the body, soothing and nourishing to the lungs, high in iron, sulphur, magnesium and potassium to help balance body.

*Fennel:* contains anticonvulsive and pain-relieving properties, eliminates mucus, soothes the nerves, helps in digestion, coughs and bronchitis.

## HERBAL COMBINATION NO. 3

*Ginger:* settles upset stomach and indigestion, helps to fight off colds, flu and fevers. Removes congestion, relieves headaches, aches and pains and helps clear throat of obstructions. contains vitamins A and C, and minerals, calcium, magnesium and potassium.

*Capsicum:* great stimulant for blood circulation, increases the power of all herbs, and helps heal the stomach and intestinal tract. Rids the body of toxins while cleansing the veins and mucous membranes.

*Goldenseal:* a wonder herb, with natural antibiotic properties, cleans toxins from the liver, stomach, and intestinal tract, kills viruses and germs and speeds healing in the body.

*Licorice:* eliminates fluid from the lungs, stimulates the adrenal glands, good for the throat, coughs and the lungs, helps when under stress and eliminates toxins from the liver.

## HERBAL COMBINATION NO. 4

*Burdock:* a great blood purifier, dissolves deposits in the joints and reduces swelling, cleans the kidneys, healing properties with antibiotic and antifungal action to promote healing in colds, flu and fevers.

*Goldenseal:* contains healing properties, helps to equalize blood sugar, destroys germs and viruses, and neutralizes acids in the body for healing.

*Parsley:* very high in nutrients to speed healing, natural diuretic to clean the kidneys and bladder, and helps eliminate toxins from the blood.

*Althea:* helps to expel phlegm from the lungs and bronchial tubes, very soothing and healing to the mucous membranes, which aids in cleaning inflammation in the body.

*Ephedra:* a great bronchodilator, which relieves congestion from colds, flu, bronchitis and asthma. It protects the lungs during the winter from infections. It also increases metabolism to promote balance in the body.

*Capsicum:* stimulating to eliminate toxins from the body and promote healing. Will also protect from colds, and flu by keeping the system clean and free from toxins.

*Horehound:* natural expectorant properties to loosen hard phlegm from the lungs. Promotes healing and stimulates, bile production for better digestion.

*Yerba Santa:* stimulates and expels phlegm from the lungs and bronchial tubes, cleans liver and stomach, clean mucous from the sinuses, helps clear the liver and stomach of mucous.

## OTHER USES

| | |
|---|---|
| Bronchitis | Childhood Diseases |
| Ear Infection | Fevers |
| Flu | General Infection |
| Mucus | Viral Infection |
| Tonsillitis | |

## SPECIAL DIETARY AIDS

*Vitamin A:* heals infections, high amounts for a few days
*Vitamin B6:* important in protein and carbohydrate metabolism
*Bioflavonoids:* necessary for healthy capillaries
*Vitamin C:* to fight infection, increases resistance
*Vitamin D:* improves absorption of calcium and phosphorus
*Vitamin E:* reduces uric acid
*Calcium:* builds blood, sustains nerves
*Rutin:* works with vitamin C for healing capillaries
*Fruits, Fresh (Juices):* for a few days, germs are burned up and eliminated and mucus will be eliminated from the lungs
*Green Drinks:* cleans and deodorizes the whole system
*Juice:* hot lemon with honey will help open the pores and sweat
*Soup, Vegetable Broth:* builds the body (use every few hours)
*Water, Pure:* cleans the body
*Whey Drinks:* contain Lysine and quality protein, contain lactose which increases utilization of calcium magnesium, and phosphorus

## ORTHODOX PRESCRIBED MEDICATION

### PSEUDOEPHEDRINE

Pseudoephedrine is prescribed for the relief of nasal congestion caused by colds, allergies and related conditions. High doses can cause these side effects:

| | |
|---|---|
| Irregular heartbeat | Hay fever |
| Hallucinations | Seizures |
| Nervousness | Restlessness |
| Trouble in sleeping | Difficult or painful urination |
| Dizziness or light-headedness | Headache |
| Nausea or vomiting | Trembling |
| Troubled breathing | Weakness |

## HYDROCODONE/TUSSEND

This combination is used to relieve coughing, reduce nasal congestion, and loosen mucus and phlegm in the lungs. Its common side effects include:

| | |
|---|---|
| Dizziness | Drowsiness |
| Feeling faint | Light-headedness |
| Nausea or vomiting | Nervousness |
| Restlessness | Trouble in sleeping |
| Constipation | Diarrhea |
| Difficult or painful urination | Headache |
| Stomach pain | Trembling |

# COLITIS

*I*nflammatory diseases of the colon, such as ulcerative colitis, amoebic colitis and bacillary dysentery. In the early stage there is abdominal cramps or pain, diarrhea and rectal bleeding. Instead of being absorbed by the body, water and minerals are rapidly expelled through lower digestive tract, which can cause dehydration or anemia. The cause of the disease is unknown, although there is a connection between colitis and depression or anxiety. A healthy colon is necessary for a healthy body. When the colon is healthy, waste is removed quickly. Proper rest, exercise, emotional health, and a healthy diet is necessary for a healthy colon. A sluggish colon could be due to improperly assimilated foods, poor eating habits, lack of exercise, lack of relaxation and emotional disturbances.

Colitis is seen as an allergic reaction, probably caused from a leaky gut syndrome. This causes the intestinal tract to become irritated from certain food and allow undigested food to enter the bloodstream and causes allergic reaction in the colon.

Digestive enzymes need to be introduced to help break up the undigested protein in the blood. If taken between meals, some will get in the blood stream. A natural product from the Morinda plant will also provide enzymes to heal and break up the undigested material and eliminate it from the body.

## HERBAL COMBINATION NO. 1

*Marshmallow:* contains mucilage that aids the bowels, very healing

*Slippery Elm:* soothes, draws out impurities, heals and acts as a buffer against irritations

*Ginger:* helps hold together all herbs, relieves gas, settles stomach

*Wild Yam:* relaxes the muscles of the stomach, and acts as sedative on the bowels

*Dong Quai:* stimulates production of interferon to help fight infections, contains antibacterial and antifungal properties, purifiers blood and improves circulation.

## OTHER USES

| | |
|---|---|
| Indigestion | Stomach Upset |
| Colon, Irritable | Intestinal Mucus |
| Diarrhea | Bowel Problems |

## SPECIAL DIETARY AIDS

*Aloe Vera:* very healing for the intestinal tract

*Hydrochloric Acid:* essential to use with protein to assure of proper digestion and assimilation

*Glucosamine Sulfate:* protects the mucous membranes and helps in healing

*Free-Form Amino Acids:* necessary for healing the intestinal tract

*Essential Fatty Acids:* necessary for healing the mucous membranes, healing for the glands, to help in the production of enzymes

*Vitamins A, E, And B-Complex:* A heals infections, B helps restore strength to the body, C fights infections, and E helps eliminate poisons in the body

*Vitamin K:* cold pressed oil

*Vitamin F:* to restore worn-down tissues

*Calcium:* dolomite, calms the nerves

*Iron:* to help avoid anemia

*Magnesium:* creates a good disposition

*Acidophilus:* produces friendly bacteria in small intestines

*Buttermilk:* coats and soothes the stomach and colon, produces friendly bacteria in colon

*Comfrey:* soothing to the tissues, settles the stomach, aids absorption of iron

*Fasting:* can help inflammation disappear and tissues heal

*Figs:* dried or tree ripened, they work upon the glands, gently prompting them by giving an emollient effect on the intestines and help bring about intestinal regularity

*Juice, Fresh Orange:* provides vitamin C, nourishing

*Kefir:* drink similar to yogurt, nourishing

*Kelp:* helps nourish the glands

*Millet:* nourishing and soothing to the digestive tract

*Papaya:* aids digestion, nourish the body

*Pepsin:* soothing to the tissues, settles the stomach

*Raw Foods:* should be blended until condition heals

*Rice, Brown:* nourishing and easily assimilated

*Sprouts:* use often when colon is healed, they act as an intestinal broom to keep waste matter moving along the intestinal tract

*Vegetables, Whole:* when colon is healed

*Wheat, Whole Bread:* helps eliminate diarrhea, provides vitamins and minerals

*Yogurt:* introduces friendly bacteria into the stomach, soothing to the colon

*Uncooked Foods:* helps prevent accumulation of colon pockets, provide bulk for diet, and prevent putrefactive fermentation.

## ORTHODOX PRESCRIBED MEDICATION

### SULFASALAZINE

Sulfasalazine is a sulfa medicine. It is given to help control inflammatory bowel disease such as colitis. Its common side effects include:

| | |
|---|---|
| Diarrhea | Dizziness |
| Headache | Itching |
| Loss of appetite | Nausea |
| Sunlight sensitivity | Rash |
| Vomiting | Aching of joints and muscles |
| Difficulty in swallowing | Pale skin |
| Unexplained sore throat/fever | Unusual bleeding or bruising |
| Unusual fatigue/weakness | Yellowing of eyes or skin |

# ENERGY

*L*ack of energy seems to be an epidemic in America. Poor eating habits and lack of exercise are the chief causes. Fatigue could be a symptom of many illnesses. One should seek for good nutrition, exercise and adequate rest. Overeating is also a cause of lack of energy, especially white sugar products in the diet.

## HERBAL COMBINATION NO. 1

*Siberian Ginseng:* natural adaptogen properties to help the body deal with stress, improves circulation and mental alertness, cleans and nourishes the body.

*Bee Pollen:* contains balanced nutrients to nourish the mind and body, contains vitamins, minerals, amino acids, fats, and enzymes.

*Yellow Dock:* cleanses the blood, liver and lymphatic system, rich in iron,vitamins A and C. It stimulates elimination, improving flow of bile and acting as a laxative.

*Licorice:* stimulates the adrenal glands to increase energy, it helps in inflammation of the intestinal tract helping to nourish and cleanse the stomach. Contains natural interferon properties to strengthen and protect the immune system.

*Gotu Kola:* can rebuild and strengthen the brain and nervous system, it combats stress, relieves high blood pressure, mental fatigue, senility, ADD, and can help in memory retention and learning problems. It is considered food for the brain.

*Kelp:* very rich in minerals to help in brain function. Good for the glands, regulates the metabolism to burn up excess calories, Strengthens the nervous system as well as the brain.

*Schizandra:* protects the body from stress with its adaptogen properties, strengthens the nervous system and the brain, protects against free radical damage. It helps to balance the body and protect against disease.

*Barley Grass:* rich in nutrients to cleanse the blood and improve the immune system, it cleans and nourishes the intestinal tract for proper digestion and assimilation. Supplies B12, so necessary for energy. It is very rich in vitamin C, and minerals to protect the body from disease and free radical damage.

*Rose Hips:* very high in vitamin C and bioflavonoids to prevent infections, strengthens the immune system. It cleans the blood and veins, and strengthens and protects the brain from damage.

*Capsicum:* speeds up chemical reaction of herbs in this formula, equalizes blood pressure, cleans and nourishes the veins and capillaries, for healthy eyes, ears and brain.

## OTHER USES

| | |
|---|---|
| Drug Withdrawal | Endurance |
| Fatigue | Longevity |
| Memory | Senility |

## SPECIAL DIETARY AIDS

*Essential Fatty Acids:* necessary for healthy glands, protects the brain and nervous system against fatigue.

*Hydrochloric Acid:* necessary for the digestion of protein to prevent allergies. Protein is essential for healing the brain and nervous system.

*Digestive Enzymes:* protects the glands from damage and the immune system. Enzymes are necessary for every function of the body.

*Vitamin B-complex:* especially B12 deficiency will cause abnormal fatigue, helps thinking

*Biotin:* promotes mental health

*Vitamin C:* decreases the probability of blood vessel rupture and stroke, increases the aging person's ability to withstand the stress of injury and infections

*Vitamin D:* necessary in tissue cell respiration and it is essential to maintain a normal basal metabolism

*Vitamin E:* increases production of hormones and reduces uric acid; promotes the functions of the sexual glands

*Iodine:* helps thyroid produce thyroxin, which is vital to mental energy

*Iron:* enriches the blood, helps clear thinking

*Almonds:* high in protein and B-complex for energy

*Bee Pollen:* contains all essential nutrients for a healthy body

*Brewer's Yeast:* contains B-complex, which is the best source of enzyme-producing compounds

*Energy Drink:* blend sunflower seeds, dates and 1 cup pure water

*Juice:* tomato or vegetable with Brewer's yeast and tea, kelp added as a pep-up drink

*Seeds, Sunflower:* protein and B-complex for energy

*Vegetable Protein:* any kind will help energy

*Watercress:* high in vitamin E and iodine, helps stimulate the brain

## ORTHODOX PRESCRIBED MEDICATION

### CAFFEINE

Caffeine stimulates the heart, brain and nervous system, depletes vitamins in the body, especially vitamin B, and also destroys vitamin A, iron and potassium. The caffeal content destroys the pepsin of the stomach and interferes with digestion of food and the absorption of food from the intestines. Caffeine is an alkaloid, a vegetable poison. It is a potent central nervous system stimulant. It may lead to headache, tremors, nervousness and irritability. Many people take coffee for energy. It is not necessarily prescribed by doctors, but they usually don't discourage the use of it.

# EYE PROBLEMS

*E*ye problems include cataracts, iridocyclitis, conjunctivitis, weak eyes and night blindness. Conjunctivitis is an infection of the mucous membrane that lines the eyelids. Symptoms include redness, swelling, itching and pus in the membrane. This could be caused by allergy, bacteria, virus, and air pollution. The following formula can be used as an eye wash.

## HERB COMBINATION NO. 1

*Goldenseal:* natural antibiotic for eye infections, kills poison
*Bayberry:* high in vitamin C, kills germs, stimulating to mucous membranes
*Eyebright:* healing, and strengthens immunity to eye complaints

## OTHER USES

| | |
|---|---|
| Air Pollution | Eye Wash |
| Allergies | Cataracts |

Diabetes
Hay Fever
Vision (Improves)

Eye Inflammation
Itching

## SPECIAL DIETARY AIDS

*Bilberry:* contains antiseptic and nutritive properties. Improves circulation in the little capillaries in the eye area, can help to sharpen vision, eye fatigue, eye irritations, night blindness, and nearsightedness.

*Vitamin A:* aids in vision and healthy eyes

*Vitamin B-complex:* especially B6, helps prevent infection of eyes

*Calcium:* helps in preventing cataracts

*Vitamin C:* detoxifying agent, heals infections

*Vitamin D:* works with Vitamin A for healthy eyes

*Vitamin E:* used with Vitamin A to help activate each other

*Cleansing Diet:* would help improve the system and may help strengthen the eyes

*Juices, Fresh Fruit:* for severe days along with pure water to keep the bowels clear

*Apples, Blueberries, Coconuts:* good for weak eyes

*Fresh Carrot Juice:* diluted with pure water, high in vitamin A for healthy eyes

*Raw Potato Juice:* said to improve eyes

*Sunflower Seeds:* nourishing to the eyes, especially for weak eyes

*Vegetables Good For Weak Eyes:* beets, broccoli, cabbage, carrots, onion, turnip, collards, leaf lettuce, and watercress.

# FASTING

Juice fasting helps control hunger, and helps keep blood sugar level normal while fasting. Fasting helps when we need to cleanse toxins from our body. We should eliminate mucus forming foods from our diet. Substitute herbs instead of using prescription drugs. Fasting helps the body, physically, spiritually and mentally.

## HERB COMBINATION NO. 1

*Licorice:* good for strength and quick energy, nourishes glands, inhibits growth of harmful viruses

*Hawthorne:* burns up excess fat in the body, strengthens heart, helps insomnia, calms nervous system

*Fennel:* internal anesthetic, useful for gas, cramps, and mucus accumulations

*Beet:* stimulates and cleans the liver, nutritious, strengthens the system

## SPECIAL DIETARY AIDS

*Essential Fatty Acids:* necessary nutrients missing in the American diet, nourishes the glands, are needed for every function of the body.

*Digestive Enzymes:* will help the body digest food better and to also break down undigested protein that can build up in the bloodstream.

*B-Complex Vitamins:* provide the body with energy, converting carbohydrates into glucose which the body burns to produce energy

*Green Drinks:* cleans the blood of impurities

*Juice, Fruits:* will flush impurities, contains minerals which contain alkalines to balance the acids which are in large quantity in the blood and tissues. It will cleanse the system of impurities

*Juices, Vegetables:* a raw vegetable juice fast to cleanse out the system of toxic debris and restore the glands to health

*Vegetable Broth:* seasoned with herbs, high in potassium which is needed for keeping the chemical balance of the fluids in the cells.

## ORTHODOX PRESCRIBED MEDICATION

Sometimes water fasting is recommended. Too long a water fast can be harmful, as it removes toxic waste too fast from the system and thickens the blood to put a strain on the heart and arteries. A juice fast is much safer. It helps keep the blood stream clean, contains alkaline and helps the tissues get plenty of oxygen, and keeps the bowels clean. Light exercise is important while fasting.

# FEMALE PROBLEMS

Recent studies have revealed that premenstrual tension is increased because of a lack of good nutrition and exercise. A good diet and exercise along with wise use of herbs would help alleviate the discomforts of menopause, menstrual problems, pregnancy and premenstrual tension. Severe cramping during menstrual cycle could be caused by hormone imbalance. It is important to be checked by your doctor to determine any serious problems. Herbs can play an important part in female problems, whether it is cramps, menopause, premenstrual tension, uterine infections or pregnancy. Red raspberry is in all the following combinations and is excellent for all female problems.

## HERBAL COMBINATION NO. 1

*Goldenseal:* kills infection, internal antiseptic, reduces swelling
*Red Raspberry:* high in iron, cleanses breasts for pure milk, regulates muscles in uterine contractions
*Black Cohosh:* natural estrogen, good relaxant in hysteria, neutralizes uric acid buildup
*Queen of the Meadow:* diuretic properties, soothes nerves helping pain in uterus
*Ginger:* distributes herbs, good for suppressed menstruation

*Marshmallow:* high in calcium, healing mucous membranes, good for menstrual problems

*Blessed Thistle:* helps lactation, good for headaches, menstrual pains, stops excessive bleeding

*Capsicum:* stimulates other herbs to do their job

*Dong Quai:* relaxes the nervous system, relieves menstrual problems, feeds the female glands, cleanses and purifies the blood and liver of "bad" estrogen.

## HERBAL COMBINATION NO. 2

*Red Raspberry:* strengthens walls of uterus, settles nausea, prevents hemorrhage

*Dong Quai:* tranquilizes central nervous system, regulates menstruating, nourishes female glands

*Ginger:* holds herbs together, stimulating to circulation, healing properties

*Licorice:* contains female estrogen, stimulates the adrenal glands, supplies energy

*Queen of the Meadow:* helps in uterine pain, diuretic, antiseptic to system

*Blessed Thistle:* internal cleanser, digestive aid, tonic to system

*Marshmallow:* heals inflammations and prevents infections, tranquilizing system

## HERBAL COMBINATION NO. 3

*Goldenseal:* reduces swelling, kills infections, eliminates toxins

*Capsicum:* equalizes blood circulation, helps distribute herbs to where they are needed

*False Unicorn:* useful for uterine disorders, promotes delayed menstruation, relieves depression

*Ginger:* binds herbs together, stimulates system, good for intestinal gas

*Uva Ursi:* increases flow of urine, good for bladder and kidney infections

*Cramp Bark:* helpful for severe menstrual or labor pains, regulates pulse, and soothing to the nerves

*Squaw Vine:* antiseptic for vaginal infections, helps morning sickness, eliminates excess toxins

*Blessed Thistle:* useful for painful menstruation, helps in headaches due to female problems

*Red Raspberry:* helps reduce hot flashes, morning sickness, cramps, strengthens uterus

## OTHER USES

| | |
|---|---|
| Breast Problems | Cramps |
| Hormone Balance | Hot Flashes |
| Hysterectomy | Menopause |
| Menstrual Problems | Morning Sickness |
| Sterility | Uterine Infections |
| Vaginal Problems | |

## SPECIAL DIETARY AIDS

*Wild Yam Cream:* useful to help balance hormones, supplies progesterone to balance estrogen, relieves menstrual problems, menopausal symptoms, helps in depression.

*Vitamin A:* necessary in pregnancy and lactation, protects the body from infections and also promotes digestion

*Vitamin B-complex:* especially pantothenic acid and PABA, help relieve nervous irritability. Brewer's Yeast supplements the lack of estrogen in the body due to various ingredients; especially needed during the middle years relieving the tension of all glands and nerves

*Herbal Calcium Formula:* rich in silicon and calcium, and minerals to help in calcium assimilation. Help to aid in the elimination of excess estrogen, and prevent bone loss, eases cramps.Vitamin B helps to prevent aging prematurely, protects the muscle of the heart; very good for improving the circulation

*Vitamin B6:* decreases anxiety, heart palpitations, perspiration, and flashes and increases ability to cope with stress, especially in premenstrual tension and eases menstrual cramps. More energy. This vitamin stimulates the production of dopamine a cerebral hormone which has a calming effect on the nervous system. Should be taken during premenstrual week and during menstruation

*Vitamin C:* helps in preventing heart attacks, assists in removing cholesterol from the body, blood vessels are strengthened, helps absorb iron, formation of red blood cells

*Vitamin D:* great effect on the reproductive organs, important in preventing miscarriages and increases fertility

*Vitamin E:* has a reducing effect on nervous sweating and at the same time relaxing the sympathetic nervous system when taken with unsaturated fatty acids (cold pressed oils) and with iron helps to form hemoglobin rich blood cells to counteract the depletion of estrogen in the body during menopause

*Iron:* helps prevent anemia

*Kelp:* help avoid anemia during menstrual flow. Helps the thyroid gland and helps control obesity in menopause

*Manganese:* helps in maintaining strong nerve health, helps to promote milk in pregnancy; resistance to disease, protects inside lining of the heart and blood vessels, increases activity of glandular system and assists in maintaining normal reproductive processes

*Zinc:* has effect on entire hormonal system, helps to absorb B complex vitamins

*Fresh Raw Fruits And Vegetables:* contain a quantity of hormone-like bioflavonoids which help to heal capillaries, enrich blood vessels, and help to ease leg cramps

## ORTHODOX PRESCRIBED MEDICATION

### PREMARIN

Premarin is used to reduce menopause symptoms. Prolonged use can cause uterine and breast cancer and blood clots. The common side effects are:

| | |
|---|---|
| Cramps | Blood pressure (increases) |
| Breasts (soreness) | Breasts (lumps) |
| Eyes (yellowing) | Mental depression |
| Nausea | Skin rash |
| Swelling of ankles and feet | Vaginal discharge |

# FITNESS

*F*itness denotes a physical state of overall good health, of having the necessary energy and stamina to withstand sickness and physical and mental stressors. Exercise is very important, for it increases your capability to handle more work. It increases your heart and lung capacity and improves your mental attitude.

## HERBAL COMBINATION NO. 1

*Siberian Ginseng:* stabilizes blood pressure, good for mental anxiety and nerves

*Ho Shou Wu:* builds stamina and resistance to disease, tonic for endocrine glands

*Black Walnut:* burns up excessive toxins and fatty material, balances sugar levels

*Licorice:* stimulant for adrenal glands, supplies energy when needed, helps to maintain sugar levels

*Gentian:* high in iron, strengthens the system, stimulates the circulation, aids digestion

*Fennel:* helps stabilize the nervous system and acts as an internal anesthetic

*Bee Pollen:* strengthens and builds the system, increases work capacity, an energizing food, helps build resistance to stress and colds, influences the adrenal hormones, athletes claim championship performances

*Bayberry:* rejuvenates the adrenal glands, cleans the blood stream, removes waste

*Myrrh:* gives vitality and strength to the digestive system, a cleansing and healing herb

*Peppermint:* sedative to the stomach, strengthens the bowels, aids digestion

*Safflower:* removes hard phlegm from the system, good for the liver and gallbladder

*Eucalyptus:* antiseptic properties, potent but safe, purifies

*Lemon Grass:* stimulates heart, calms nerves, tightening action on tissues

*Capsicum:* stimulates the system, disinfectant to body, equalizes blood circulation

## OTHER USES

| | |
|---|---|
| Diets | Endurance |
| Energy | Fasting |
| Glands | Strength |

## SPECIAL DIETARY AIDS

*Vitamin B-complex:* especially B1, B3, B6, and B12. Thiamine depletion is caused by excessive amounts of sugar, smoking and alcohol, B3 works in the enzymatic breakdown of sugar in the body's energy cycle

*Vitamin C:* for stress and alertness, helps in fatigue

*Vitamin E:* improves stamina and lung control of oxygen

*Amino Acids, Essential:* necessary to healthy cells in the body
*Magnesium:* essential for effective nerve and muscle function
*Bee Pollen:* increases endurance
*Brewer's Yeast:* concentrated live food with B vitamins and protein, increases the action of vitamin E
*Fruits:* increases energy, apricots, cantaloupe, guava, papayas, peaches

## ORTHODOX PRESCRIBED MEDICATION

### AMPHETAMINES

Benzedrine and Methadrine, often called "uppers" and "pep pills," have been used by athletes and diet-conscious persons. It increases heart rate, blood sugar, muscle tension, and gives a sense of well-being. The extra energy is borrowed from the body's reserves. When the drug's action has worn off, the body pays for it in fatigue and depression. This creates the desire for more of the drug. Its possible side effects include:

Psychic dependence                 Physical deterioration
Psychotic paranoia/schizophrenia

# GLANDS

All glands are vital to a healthy system. They need to be nourished especially with minerals. Vitamins and minerals play an important part in supplying the body with the raw material to manufacture its own hormones which are the secretions of the glands. These hormones are essential secretions affecting the whole system, and are connected with growth and health. The glands depend on the necessary intake of the vital vitamins and minerals for their efficient functioning. The thyroid gland stimulates all of the cells of the body. The hormones from the thyroid are powerful and need to be kept under exact control. Lack of iodine is a common cause of trouble. Diseases or drugs can effect the thyroid, also stress or hereditary defect.

## HERBAL COMBINATION NO. 1

*Kelp:* contains iodine which strengthens and reactivates the glands, strengthens blood and central nervous system
*Dandelion:* stimulates glands, increases activity of liver, tonic, nutritious
*Alfalfa:* increases glandular secretions, nourishes glands

## HERBAL COMBINATION NO. 2

*Licorice:* nourishes the adrenal glands, stimulates interferon production to protect the immune system.
*Lemon Bioflavonoids:* strengthens the veins and glands
*Asparagus Powder:* rich in nutrients to nourish glands
*Alfalfa:* rich in minerals and vitamins to nourish the glands, especially the pituitary.
*Parsley:* natural diuretic, rich in essential minerals
*Black Walnut:* high in iodine which kills toxins, candida, parasites and worms.
*Thyme:* antiseptic properties to remove toxins from the glands.
*Parthenium:* cleans blood and lymphatic congestion.
*Schizandra:* contains properties to strengthen the body, increases energy, protects against free radical damage.
*Siberian Ginseng:* increases circulation, mental alertness, nourishes the glands, cleans the blood and veins.
*Dong Quai:* cleans and purifies blood, balances hormones, calms nerves, feeds the glands.
*Dandelion:* cleans and nourishes the liver, helps to eliminate excess hormones from the liver, rich in vitamin A and potassium.

*Uva Ursi:* tonic for the pancreas and other glands, natural diuretic, strong antibiotic properties.

*Marshmallow:* soothing and healing for the digestive, and intestinal tract, tonic properties, nutritive.

*Beta Carotene:* necessary for healthy glands, prevents infections, builds up the immune system.

*Vitamin C:* nourishing for the glands, prevents infections, strengthens the immune system.

*Vitamin E and Zinc:* work together to an antioxidant, protects the immune system, necessary for glandular health.

*Pantothenic Acid:* antistress nutrient to nourish the adrenal glands. Helps protect the body against stress and injury.

*Manganese:* necessary for proper functioning of nerves, involved in enzymes function of nutrients, necessary for strong bones, cartilage and skin.

*Potassium:* necessary for healthy veins and heart, works with sodium for acid-alkaline balance, prevents glandular problems.

*Lecithin:* necessary for nerve health, prevents fat accumulation in the liver and veins.

## OTHER USES

| | |
|---|---|
| Asthma | Pets (Vitamins And Minerals) |
| Breasts | Bronchitis |
| Croup | Liver |
| Lymph Congestion | Mucus |
| Nerves | Pain |
| Pituitary | Pleurisy |
| Pneumonia | Rheumatism |
| Thyroid | Tonsillitis |

## SPECIAL DIETARY AIDS

*Vitamin A:* healing vitamin, rejuvenates the glands, repairs damaged tissues

*Vitamin B-complex:* necessary for metabolism of the extra carbohydrates and protein, helps replenish nutrition to glands

*Vitamin C:* healing vitamin, protects the glands, helps glands to become nutritionally replenished

*Vitamin E:* increases production of hormones

*Calcium:* assists all metabolic functions to perform efficiently

*Chlorine:* acts in formation of glandular hormones, helps in metabolism

*Iodine:* aids thyroid gland, promotes metabolism, prevents goiter

*Iron:* nourishes the glands

*Magnesium:* stimulates the glands

*Manganese:* increases gland secretion

*Phosphorus:* promotes secretion of hormones

*Potassium:* increases glandular secretions

*Silicon:* stimulates and feeds the glands

*Zinc:* necessary for synthesis of new body protein

*Alfalfa Sprouts:* full of enzymes, nourishing to the glands

*Avocado:* gland food, use with olive oil

*Broccoli:* feeds weak glands involved in digestion of food

*Dates:* nourishing food for glands

*Figs (Tree: Ripened):* medicine for the glands, supplies nutrients

*Fluids:* fresh pure water, fresh fruit and vegetable juices

*Nuts, Raw Almond And Cashew:* supplies protein, needed daily for the cells

*Olive Oil:* lubricates the system, supplies vitamins

*Parsley:* cleans the glands, nourishes

*Protein (Not Red Meat):* to replace muscle tissue and build cells

*Raisins:* nourishes the glands

*Rice And Bran:* feeds the glands and cells

*Rye:* good for the glands, high in protein

*Seeds:* pumpkin, squash, sunflower, and sesame, seeds are gland foods

*Yams:* gland food

## ORTHODOX PRESCRIBED MEDICATION

### LIOTRIX OR THYROGLOBULIN

These are typical thyroid hormones prescribed for thyroid function. Their possible side effects include:

| | |
|---|---|
| Constipation | Chest pain |
| Hives | Listlessness |
| Muscle aches | Rapid pulse |
| Shortness of breath | Fatigue |

# HEART

*H*eart attacks are the leading cause of death in the U.S. Many Americans have coronary artery disease, which is characterized by a narrowing of the blood vessels that nourish the heart muscle. The narrowing of the vital coronary vessels may progress for many years before any adverse effects are evident. In many instances a heart attack is the first overt sign of the disease.

## HERBAL COMBINATION NO. 1

*Hawthorn:* strengthens the heart, helps prevent blood clot near heart, high in minerals
*Capsicum:* takes other herbs to the heart, circulation
*Garlic:* kills infection, heart palpitation, lowers blood pressure, beneficial to blood vessels

## HERBAL COMBINATION NO. 2

*Ginkgo:* supplies oxygen and nutrition to the heart and veins, aids in arterial blood flow, senility, vertigo, tinnitus, depression, memory, and intermittent claudication.

*Hawthorn:* nourishes and strengthens the heart, useful in rapid and feeble heart action, heart valve defects, enlarged heart, angina pectoris and lack of oxygen in the blood.

## HERBAL COMBINATION NO. 3

*Capsicum:* increases circulation to the heart and veins, rebuilds tissues, heals stomach and intestinal tract.

*Hawthorn:* strengthens the heart, cleans the veins, protects against toxin accumulating in the blood.

*Coenzyme Q-10:* supplies oxygen in the blood to improve heart function. Helps increase energy and brain function.

*Copper:* necessary for iron absorption, is involved in the metabolism of vitamin C, involved in myelin sheath health, builds bone and collagen health.

*Iron:* responsible for carrying oxygen from the lungs to all parts of the body. Vital for a healthy immune system.

*Magnesium:* important in maintaining healthy nerves, relaxes the muscles, including the heart.

*Zinc:* essential for cell division, cell repair and growth. Necessary for a healthy appetite.

*Histidine:* an essential amino acid which nourishes the brain, protects the immune system and protects against allergies.

*Glycine:* rids the body of waste material, and protect against toxic build-up.

## OTHER USES

| | |
|---|---|
| Adrenal | Arteriosclerosis |
| Anxiety | Circulation |
| Cholesterol | Fatigue |
| Hardening Of Arteries | Irregular Heart Beat |
| Liver | Pain |
| Shock | Varicose Veins |

## SPECIAL DIETARY AIDS

*Vitamin B-complex:* especially B1, B12, necessary to maintain the health of the arteries

*Vitamin C:* nourishes the capillaries

*Vitamin D:* relaxes nerves, helps calcium absorb

*Vitamin E:* needed as an anticoagulant to reduce arterial clots and to get oxygen to the blood

*Vitamin F:* increases circulation

*Vitamin K:* aids blood coagulation and controls consistency of blood

*Calcium:* calms nerves, strengthens heart muscles

*Lecithin:* helps eliminate cholesterol

*Magnesium:* alkalizes the system, aids blood circulation

*Phosphorus:* helps in acid, alkaline balance

*Potassium:* vital in preventing heart attacks (combined with magnesium)

*Diet, Cleansing:* to clean out the arteries

*Fruits, Fresh:* live enzymes, vitamins and minerals to nourish the heart

*Grains, Whole:* contains B-complex vitamin, minerals, enzymes and amino acids to the gland which helps to maintain a healthful blood cholesterol level. The hormones feed the heart muscles to send oxygen to the circulatory system

*Oils, Cold Pressed:* it sends a natural antioxidant hormone to the heart and boosts the heart-blood circulation

*Protein:* vegetable is better quality, does not leave uric acid build-up. Use honey, pure maple syrup, malt sugar, date sugar instead of white sugar.

*Olives:* rich in potassium

*Potassium "Soup":* potato peelings, celery, onions, carrots, parsley. Cook and strain

## ORTHODOX PRESCRIBED MEDICATION

### NITROGLYCERIN

Nitroglycerin is prescribed to improve the supply of blood and oxygen to the heart. It also relieves pain and/or prevents heart attacks. Its possible side effects include:

| | |
|---|---|
| Headache | Dizziness |
| Flushing | Nausea |
| Skin Rash | Vomiting |
| Weakness | |

### PROCAINAMIDE

This is prescribed to restore irregular heartbeats to a normal rhythm and to slow an overactive heart. Its possible side effects include:

| | |
|---|---|
| Diarrhea | Loss of appetite |
| Nausea | Vomiting |
| Fever | Itching |
| Joint pain or swelling | Pains with breathing |
| Skin rash | Mental confusion |
| Mental depression | Hallucinations |
| Unexplained fever/sore throat | Unusual bleeding or bruising |

# HIGH BLOOD PRESSURE

*H*ypertension is a condition in which the person has a higher blood pressure than is judged to be normal. High blood pressure is the body's extensive measure to cope with functions of the body, such as toxemia, kidney problems, glandular disturbances, degenerative changes in arteries, overweight or emotional problems. With high blood pressure, there is a thickening of the blood from catarrhal and excess matter loading the circulatory system. High blood pressure is usually characterized by flushed complexion, overweight, and discomfort. Some doctors feel it is a result of improper living habits which cause a run-down condition of the body. High and low blood pressure are both due to malfunction of the circulatory system. Cholesterol must be eliminated from the system to help the blood to flow more easily. Stress is a factor in causing high blood pressure and should be controlled.

## HERBAL COMBINATION NO. 1

*Hawthorn:* regulates blood pressure whether high or low, strengthens the heart and veins, nourishes the heart and blood.
*Capsicum:* stimulates the system and the ingredient of garlic reduces the dilated blood vessels
*Garlic:* antibiotic, opens up the blood vessels and reduces blood pressure in hypertension

## HERBAL COMBINATION NO. 2

*Garlic:* helps stabilize blood pressure, purifies the system
*Capsicum:* carries the herbs where needed, natural stimulant
*Parsley:* high in iron, natural diuretic, helps resist infection
*Ginger:* helps bind the herbs together, removes excess waste
*Siberian Ginseng:* stabilizes blood pressure, hormone regulator
*Goldenseal:* antiseptic, cleans any infection, controls secretions

## OTHER USES

| | |
|---|---|
| Circulation | Colds |
| Flu | High Blood Pressure |
| Hypertension | Infections |
| Low Blood Pressure | Nerves |
| Stress | Tension |

## SPECIAL DIETARY AIDS

*Vitamin A:* builds the immune system

*Vitamin B-complex:* high potency, calms the nerves and helps build the blood

*Vitamin C:* strengthens the blood vessels

*Vitamin E:* dilates the blood vessels, could temporarily elevate blood pressure, small amount to start

*Bioflavonoids:* helps maintain the health of the blood vessels

*Calcium:* a deficiency has been found to be a major cause of high blood pressure

*Choline:* prevents fats from accumulating in the liver and assists the movement of fats into the cells

*Magnesium:* helps the nervous system and promotes sleep

*Lecithin:* breaks up cholesterol and allows it to pass through the arterial wall, helping to prevent arteriosclerosis

*Manganese:* necessary for proper nutrition, activates other minerals

*Potassium:* will cause the body to excrete more sodium

*Rutin:* to strengthen capillaries

*Sulphur:* promotes bile secretions, purifies the system

*Tyrosine (Natural Amino Acid):* experiments in Israel have shown to help reverse high blood pressure

*Zinc:* influences acid: alkaline balance in body

*Broccoli:* good for high blood pressure

*Buckwheat:* complete protein equal to animal protein

*Cantaloupe:* full of vitamins and minerals, has been recommended for high blood pressure

*Rice And Fruit:* recommended to help clear out the system

*Exercise:* is important to keep the circulation system healthy

*Garlic:* contains sulphur and manganese, helps cholesterol and cleans the blood vessels

*Parsley:* natural diuretic, full of vitamins and minerals

*Pineapple:* regulates the glands, is valuable for high blood pressure

*Rice, Wild:* high in vitamins and minerals and low in fat

*Strawberries:* cleans the blood of harmful toxins

*Tea, Taheebo:* cleans the blood, strengthens the body

*Tomatoes:* natural antiseptic and protects against infection, helps in high blood pressure

*Watermelon:* cleans out the system. The seeds contain cucurbocitrin, which dilates the capillaries, the tiny blood vessels. This relieves pressure on the large blood vessels.

## ORTHODOX PRESCRIBED MEDICATION

### RESERPINE AND HYDRALAZINE

These are medicines called antihypertensives, and are prescribed to treat high blood pressure. They are also sometimes used to treat certain mental and emotional conditions. Their common side effects include:

| | |
|---|---|
| Drowsiness or fainting | General feeling of weakness |
| Headache | Decreased sexual interest |
| Mental depression | Nervousness |
| Vivid dreams or nightmares | Black, tarry stools |
| Chest pain | Bloody vomit |
| Numbness | Shortness of breath |
| Skin rash | Stiffness |

# HYPOGLYCEMIA

*H*ypoglycemia is a condition where there is a deficiency of sugar in the blood or low blood sugar, in other, words a condition in which the glucose in the blood is abnormally low. The symptoms are fatigue, restlessness, malaise, marked irritability and weakness. In severe cases, mental disturbances, delirium, coma and possibly death can occur.

## HERBAL COMBINATION NO. 1

*Licorice:* supplies quick energy to weakened systems

*Safflower:* helps the adrenal glands to produce more adrenaline and encourages the pancreas to manufacture natural insulin

*Dandelion:* destroys acids in the blood, helps in anemia, balances blood in all nutritive salts

*Horseradish:* contains antibiotic action, stimulates the system

## HERBAL COMBINATION NO. 2

*Goldenseal:* regulates blood sugar, controls uterine hemorrhaging, kills viruses, germs and parasites and worms, healing to the mucous membranes.

*Juniper Berries:* natural diuretic, contains antiseptic and antifungal properties. Cleans the blood and urinary tract.

*Uva Ursi:* helps to eliminate excess sugar in blood, natural antiseptic, cleans the liver, kidneys and bladder.

*Cedar Berries:* healing for the glands, especially the pancreas, disinfects and heals urinary tract.

*Mullein:* soothes and heals the urinary tract, pain reliever, and heals inflammations.

*Yarrow:* strengthens liver and pancreas function, controls bleeding, soothes and heals mucous membranes.

*Garlic:* natural antibiotic, cleans the blood and veins, destroys parasites which are felt to be one cause of diabetes.

*Slippery Elm:* very healing and soothing to the mucous membranes. Nourishes the blood and glands. Heals the digestive tract to improve assimilation of nutrients.

*Capsicum:* heals wounds and prevents bleeding, increases circulation, cleans blood and improves glandular activity.

*Dandelion:* rich in minerals, natural diuretic, cleans and protects the liver, cleans the blood.

*Marshmallow:* soothing for the urinary tract, cleans toxins.

*Nettle:* rich in minerals, heals and shrinks tissues, cleans blood, lymphatic system and glands.

*White Oak Bark:* astringent properties to control and stop bleeding, heals damaged tissues, glands, stomach and intestines.

*Licorice:* stimulates interferon production to protect against infections, nourishes the adrenal glands, supports all glands, cleans the liver.

## OTHER USES

| | |
|---|---|
| Adrenal Glands | Anemia |
| Energy | Liver |
| Pancreas | Weakened System |

## SPECIAL DIETARY AIDS

*Vitamin A:* gives strength and vitality, promotes healthy feeling

*Vitamin B-complex:* helps in nervous exhaustion, antistress vitamin helps normalize sugar level

*Vitamin B6:* helps build adrenal glands

*Vitamin B12:* helps restore liver function

*Vitamin C:* has been said to prevent low blood sugar attacks if taken daily

*Vitamin E:* helps in the oxygenation of cells, necessary when sugar levels are low

*Magnesium:* diabetics require more than the normal dose, necessary for the nerves

*Chromium:* is essential to the utilization of glucose

*Brewer's Yeast:* B complex to feed the cells and nerves

*Frequent Small Meals:* Provides quick energy

*Nuts:* good source of protein and unsaturated fats as well as vitamins and minerals

*Seeds:* high in protein, high in calcium and very nutritious, high in amino acid balance that enhances utilization

*Natural Carbohydrates:* needed in small quantities
*Whole Grains, Nuts, Seeds:* high quality protein
*Vegetables:* fresh for enzymes, vitamins and minerals

## ORTHODOX PRESCRIBED MEDICATION

### GLUCAGON

This drug is a hormone. This is an emergency medicine to treat severe hypo glycemia. It is used by injection if the patient becomes unconscious as a result of hypoglycemia. In many cases high animal protein is recommended. This could lead to uric acid build up in the system. Side effects could cause vomiting. Glucagon is not effective for much longer than twelve hours and is only used until the patient is able to swallow liquids.

# INFECTIONS

The condition in which the body or part of it is invaded by microorganisms or virus. The symptoms of infection are those of inflammation, swelling, and soreness. To keep infections from remaining in the system, some doctors suggest encouraging perspiration, activating the kidneys, and opening the bowels, because fevers tend to dry up the bowels. Take natural laxatives and protein foods, for protein of animal origin are contraindicated in infectious disease. Also eat raw fruits and vegetable juices while fever lasts.

## HERBAL COMBINATION NO. 1

*Cat's Claw:* strengthens the immune system, treats viral infections, reduces inflammation, heals the stomach and bowels.
*Astragalus:* increases the production of interferon to protect the immune system, tonic properties to strengthen the body.

*Echinacea:* strong antibiotic properties, can be used for long periods of time without side effects, cleans toxin from the body.

## HERBAL COMBINATION NO. 2

*Parthenium:* blood cleanser, excellent for infections, cleans liver and kidneys.

*Goldenseal:* antibiotic, kills poisons in system, reduces swellings, valuable for all catarrhal conditions

*Yarrow:* blood cleanser, opens pores to permit perspiration, eliminates impurities and reduces fevers

*Capsicum:* reduces dilated blood vessels in chronic congestion, stimulant, disinfectant

## HERBAL COMBINATION NO. 3

*Goldenseal:* acts as a natural antibiotic, reduces swelling, heals mucous membranes

*Black Walnut:* burns up excess toxins, kills infections, tones up the system

*Marshmallow:* removes difficult phlegm from system, heals, soothes and neutralizes

*Parthenium:* infection fighter, resembles echinacea's properties, cleans blood, liver and kidneys

*Plantain:* neutralizes poisons, acts as a laxative, soothing to whole system

*Bugleweed:* helps reduce fluid discharges, relieves pain, relaxes the body

## OTHER USES

| | |
|---|---|
| Breasts, Infection | Colds |
| Contagious Diseases | Earache |
| Fevers | Flu |
| Gangrene | Glands, Infected, Swollen |

| | |
|---|---|
| Infections | Lungs |
| Measles | Mumps |
| Sinus Infection | Throat, Sore |
| Tonsillitis | Typhoid Fever |

## SPECIAL DIETARY AIDS

*Vitamin A:* large doses for a short period promotes healing, fights infections

*Vitamin B-complex:* infections can cause depletion of B-complex, necessary to help maintain energy

*Vitamin B6:* acts as a natural antihistamine, defends body against infections

*Vitamin C:* massive dose helps fight early infection, helps in allergy related infections

*Vitamin E:* works with vitamin A to promote healing, heals infections, removes scar tissue

*Bioflavonoids:* strengthens capillaries, helps heal infections

*Zinc:* speeds up the healing of external and internal wounds

*Broth, Vegetable:* high in potassium, builds health

*Fruits, Fresh:* helps remove impurities from the blood

*Fruits, Fresh Juices:* purifies the system, builds the body

*Water, Pure:* cleans the system of poisons

*Watercress, Wild:* eaten regularly will help build immunity to colds, catarrhs, and infectious diseases

## ORTHODOX PRESCRIBED MEDICATION

### ANTIBIOTICS

Penicillin, tetracycline or erythromycin are among the most commonly prescribed antibiotics. Their side effects include:

| | |
|---|---|
| Cramps/burning of stomach | Blood in the urine |
| Diarrhea | Hives |

Sensitivity to sunlight
Itching of rectal/genital area
Sore mouth or tongue
Vomiting

Itching
Nausea
Swelling of face and ankles

# INSOMNIA

*I*nsomnia is the inability to sleep, because it is prematurely ended or interrupted by periods of wakefulness. It could be a symptom of a disease, but it is not a disease in itself. Anxiety and pain are the most frequent causes of insomnia. Some people with ailments such as asthma or heart disease may be unable to sleep for fear of suffocation. Avoid caffeine drinks.

## HERBAL COMBINATION NO. 1

*Valerian:* relaxant, sedative, tonic, tranquilizer with refreshed feeling

*Skullcap:* feeds the nerves, controls nervous disorders, relaxes the mind

*Hops:* helps restlessness, acts as a nervine for insomnia

## HERBAL COMBINATION NO. 2

*Black Cohosh:* tonic for the central nervous system, an excellent safe sedative, prevents spasms

*Valerian:* calms the nerves, natural tranquilizer

*Capsicum:* stimulating, cleansing for the nervous system, increases effectiveness of other herbs

*Passionflower:* excellent for nervous disorders and irritability, relaxing and soothing

*Skullcap:* relieves spasms and nervous disorders, feeds and nourishes the nervous system

*Hops:* has a sedative effect on the nerves, relieves pain, reduces fevers, good for insomnia, nervous stomach

*Wood Betony:* good for headaches and nervous disorders, calming and pain reliever, cleans impurities from the blood and liver

## OTHER USES

| | |
|---|---|
| Convulsions | Headaches |
| Hyperactivity | Nerves |
| Palsy | Relaxant |

## SPECIAL DIETARY AIDS

*Vitamin B-complex:* relaxing to the nerves

*Vitamin B6:* essential for break tryptophan down into niacin

*Vitamin Bl5:* improves the body's ability to withstand stressful conditions

*Tryptophan (Essential Amino Acid):* it has been used for psychiatric problems, to induce sleep and to quiet the nervous system

*Calcium:* calms the nerves, gives strength

*Choline:* assists in transmission of nerve impulses

*Folic Acid:* metabolism of proteins

*Baths, Water:* help relax

*Exercise:* vigorous morning exercise causes the release of a hormone called prostaglandin which promotes sleep twelve hours later

*Juice, Celery:* promotes sleep

*Tea, Chamomile:* produces restful sleep, but avoid a heavy meal in the evening

## ORTHODOX PRESCRIBED MEDICATION

### PHENOBARBITAL/CARBROMAL

These are medicines known as central nervous system depressants. They are given to treat insomnia or sleeplessness.

Their possible side effects include:

| | |
|---|---|
| Dizziness | Light headedness |
| Drowsiness | Hangover effect |
| Swollen eyelids, face or lips | Unusual sore throat and fever |
| Unusual bleeding/bruising | Unusual excitement |
| Fatigue | Weakness |
| Slow heart beat | |

# KIDNEYS AND BLADDER

The function of the kidneys is to excrete urine which contains the end products of metabolism, and to help regulate the wastes, electrolyte and acid base content of the blood. Nephritis is an inflammation of the kidneys. Avoid foods that contain oxalic acid, caffeine, theobromine, and caffeal (more concentrated in decaffeinated coffee). They are irritating to the kidneys. Coffee, chocolate and excessive meat should be avoided.

## HERBAL COMBINATION NO. 1.

*Juniper Berries:* clears mucus in bladder and kidneys, strengthens nerves, high in vitamin C

*Parsley:* high in potassium, which gives muscle tone to bladder, increases flow of urine

*Uva Ursi:* beneficial for bladder and kidney infections, strengthens and tones urinary tract

*Dandelion:* very nourishing, neutralizes uric acid, opens urinary passages

*Chamomile:* tonic, soothing to the nerves, helps elimination through the kidneys

## SPECIAL DIETARY AIDS

*Vitamin A:* necessary to keep the kidneys healthy

*Vitamin B6:* important for proper functioning of the pancreas

*Vitamin C:* helps keep the kidneys healthy and in good repair

*Vitamin E:* helps clear up kidney problems

*Lecithin:* helps purify the kidneys

*Manganese:* essential for proper nutrition, activates other minerals

*Magnesium:* valuable to the nervous system

*Potassium:* stimulates the liver, converts sugar into energy

*Zinc:* has an effect on acid-alkaline balance of the system. It is necessary to keep the kidneys healthy

*Apples:* contain malic and tartaric acids, which helps keep digestion and the liver healthy

*Grapes:* the alkaline in grapes helps to decrease the acidity of the uric acid and to eliminate it from the system, thus helping the kidneys

*Juices:* cherry and apple and cranberry

*Lemon Juice:* in pure water, 1/2 lemon at a time, a natural antiseptic, destroys bacteria

*Liquids:* avoid sweet drinks like soda pop, coffee, tea, chocolate and white sugar products and starches. These could cause inflammation of the lining membranes of the kidneys.

*Parsley:* natural diuretic, rich in minerals and vitamins and is valuable for nephritis

*Pears:* helps in inflammation of the kidneys, such as nephritis

*Soup:* use asparagus, celery, spinach and parsley

*Watercress:* very high in vitamin C, has been recommended for kidney disorders

*Watermelon:* well known for correcting kidney problems, the seeds contain cucurbocitrin, which has the effect of dilating the capillaries, relieving pressure on the large blood vessels

## ORTHODOX PRESCRIBED MEDICATION

### PENICILLINS

Penicillin is often prescribed for nephritis, or kidney infections. Penicillin's possible side effects are:

| | |
|---|---|
| Hives | Itching |
| Rash | Wheezing |
| Diarrhea | Nausea |
| Vomiting | Blood in urine |
| Excess light: colored urine | Swelling of face and ankles |

# LIVER AND GALLBLADDER

The liver manufactures digestive enzymes and acts as a filter between the intestines and the heart. It helps detoxify the poisons which are taken into the system. The liver controls and regulates the quantity, the quality and the use of the foods we eat. It regulates the appetite, for in the case of hepatitis, one of the first signs is loss of appetite. The liver has a vital influence on the emotions of the body. A healthy liver will help in endurance, patience, and perseverance. A sluggish liver, with accumulated toxins can cause nausea, headaches, indigestion, loss of appetite, constipation, pain on the right side, cold sweats, and jaundice. Liver problems usually involve congestion, hepatitis, and sluggishness. The liver is a powerful detoxifying organ, breaking down toxic materials, and producing bile. The three most common liver diseases are: liver cancer, cirrhosis, and hepatitis.

## HERBAL COMBINATION NO. 1

*Black Cohosh:* calming for the nerves and cleansing for the liver and gallbladder, relaxing for the body to help increase healing.

*Red Beet:* nutritious for liver function, helps correct liver disease

*Dandelion:* stimulates the liver, detoxifies poisons, clears liver obstructions

*Parsley:* cleans liver of toxic wastes, tones the body, nutritious to build system

*Horsetail:* rich in vitamins and minerals, aids in circulation, builds and tones the body, diuretic

*Liverwort:* contains vitamin K and other nutrients important to strengthen the liver, heals damaged liver

*Birch:* natural properties for cleansing the blood, high content of vitamins and minerals

*Blessed Thistle:* general tonic to system, stimulates liver bile, purifies blood

*Angelica:* helps eliminate toxins in liver and spleen, tonic for mental and physical harmony

*Chamomile:* destroys toxins in liver, healing properties, aid for insomnia

*Gentian:* stimulates liver, high in iron, strengthens the system, aids digestion

*Goldenrod:* stimulates circulation, kidney function, strengthens system

## HERBAL COMBINATION NO. 2

*Barberry:* corrects liver secretions (causes the bile to flow more freely)

*Ginger:* works as a diffusive stimulant

*Cramp Bark:* good for congestion and hardening of the liver

*Fennel:* helps move waste material out of the body

*Peppermint:* cleans and strengthens the entire body

*Wild Yam:* good for hardening and blocking of the liver

*Catnip:* used as a tonic to strengthen the liver and gallbladder

## OTHER USES

| | |
|---|---|
| Age Spots | Cleansing |
| Gall Bladder | Kidneys |
| Pancreas | Spleen |

## SPECIAL DIETARY AIDS

*Vitamin A:* promotes digestion and food assimilation

*Vitamin B-complex:* Provides amino acids, strengthens system

*Vitamin B6:* promotes digestion and elimination

*Vitamin B15:* helps in digestion, assimilation and elimination

*Vitamin C:* detoxifying properties, heals infections

*Vitamin D:* stored in the liver for all over healthy feeling

*Vitamin E:* helps reduce uric acid

*Vitamin K:* helps liver function to properly absorb food

*Magnesium:* stimulates the liver

*Zinc:* aids digestion, helps the acid, alkaline balance

*Sulphur:* aids the liver in bile secretion

*Choline:* helps detoxify fatty and congested liver and assists liver function

*Inositol:* helps prevent gallbladder problems, helps prevent fatty liver

*Methionime:* (amino acid) necessary for liver regeneration, removes poisonous wastes from the liver and protects the liver

*Vegetables:* artichokes, cauliflower, collards, endive, green peppers, pomegranate, quince, raspberries, strawberries, and tangerines

*Fruit Juices, Fresh:* cleans the liver, strengthens the system

*Fruits:* apples, cherries, cranberries, gooseberries, plums, pomegranate, quince, raspberries, strawberries and tangerines

*Carrot Juice:* cleans and nourishes the liver

*Dandelion Tea:* cleansing for the liver

*Milk Thistle:* repairs and protects the liver, liver, spleen and gallbladder tonic, increases protein synthesis in the liver.

*Garlic:* helps detoxify bacteria in the intestines

*Grains, Beans:* protein, helps in the formation of important enzymes, hormones and disease, fighting antibodies

*Grapes:* helps liver disorders, jaundice and stimulates bile flow

*Watercress And Parsley:* relieves liver inflammation

*Olive Oil In Orange Or Lemon Juice:* helps dissolve hard bile Avoid sugar, starches, fats, eggs, cream, spices, alcohol, chocolate and caffeine drinks to bring quicker results

## ORTHODOX PRESCRIBED MEDICATION

### CHOLESTYRAMINE

Cholestyramine removes bile acids from the body, especially with liver problems, where there is too much bile acid in the body. Its common side effects include:

| | |
|---|---|
| Constipation | Severe stomach pain |
| Nausea and vomiting | Unusual loss of weight |

### KANAMYCIN

This is an antibiotic that is used to help lessen the symptoms of hepatic coma, a complication of liver disease. Its possible side effects include:

| | |
|---|---|
| Irritated mouth or rectal area | Nausea |
| Vomiting | Some loss of hearing |
| Clumsiness | Dizziness |

# LOWER BOWELS

An underactive bowel can cause toxic wastes to be absorbed through the bowel wall and into the bloodstream, which can cause them to deposit in the tissues . As toxins accumulate in the tissues, they can cause cell destruction. Other problems can arise, such as poor digestion, fatigue, poor circulation and many other ailments because of improper diet and impacted bowels.

## HERBAL COMBINATION NO. 1

*Cascara Sagrada:* restores tone to relaxed bowel, cleans and nourish system

*Buckthorn:* stimulates the bile, good for constipation, calming on gastrointestinal tract

*Licorice:* mild laxative, supplies energy, beneficial to the liver

*Capsicum:* stimulates the bowels, internal cleanser, increases the power of all the other herbs

*Ginger:* internal stimulant, holds herbs together, settles the stomach.

*Barberry:* promotes bile in liver, calming for the nerves, cleansing for the system

*Couch Grass:* antibiotic, tonic, cleans the urinary tract, diuretic

*Red Clover:* cleans mucus from the system, fights infection, high in iron and minerals

*Turkey Rhubarb:* strengthens the intestinal tract, tones the bowels, cleans and heals the entire intestinal tract, natural laxative properties.

## HERBAL COMBINATION NO. 2

*Cascara Sagrada:* stimulates the gall bladder, helps liver problems, stimulates adrenal glands

*Rhubarb:* reduces blood pressure, good for chronic diarrhea, reduces inflammations

*Dong Quai:* natural relaxer for the bowels to speed healing, has antibiotic properties, cleans and purifies the blood, natural bowel lubricant to help in congestion of the colon.

*Goldenseal:* strong antibiotic, relieves inflammations, strengthens liver, healing

*Capsicum:* increases blood circulation, distributes herbs throughout the system

*Ginger:* binds other herbs together, soothing to nervous system, helps intestinal gas

*Barberry:* strong antiseptic properties, blood cleanser, removes morbid matter from stomach and bowels

*Fennel:* relieves gas, colic and cramps, nourishes the system

*Red Raspberry:* good for stomach problems, strengthens the system, supplies nutrients

## OTHER USES

| | |
|---|---|
| Bad Breath | Bowel Discomforts |
| Cleansing | Colitis |
| Colon | Constipation |
| Croup | Diarrhea |
| Intestinal Mucus | Parasites |

## SPECIAL DIETARY AIDS

*Vitamin A:* promotes digestion and assimilation of food

*Vitamin B-complex:* to avoid depletion from the system, helps build the body's resistance to disease and gives the body energy

*Vitamin C:* protection for the whole system, protects the tissues to resist infections

*Vitamin D:* helps calcium and minerals absorb, essential to maintain a normal basal metabolism

*Vitamin E:* improves circulation and reduces uric acid, protects the body from virus

*Vitamin F:* lubricant for cells giving tone and elasticity

*Calcium:* builds blood, assists digestive ferments and checks peristaltic action

*Magnesium:* aids in prevention of constipation, alkalizes system

*Zinc:* aids digestion, assists body in absorbing B-complex vitamins

*Pure Water:* cleans the bowels

*Fresh Fruit And Vegetable Juices:* provide nutrients easily assimilated

*Yogurt:* restores friendly bacteria in system

*Kefir:* high in enzymes for healthy bowels

*Comfrey And Pepsin:* helps digest proteins

*Papaya Juice:* aids digestion relieves infections in the colon and helps break down pus and mucus reached by the juice

*Bananas:* valuable and soothing to bowels, must be ripe

*Millet:* low in starch, easily digested

*Whey Powder:* high in nutrients, helps utilize calcium, easily digested

*Protein Digestive Tablets:* helps foods to digest and soothing to the bowels, important in helping to digest meat

## ORTHODOX PRESCRIBED MEDICATION

### SULFASALAZINE

This is used to help control inflammatory bowel disease such as enteritis or colitis. Its common side effects include:

| | |
|---|---|
| Continuing headache | Sensitivity to sunlight |
| Itching | Rash |
| Aching of joints and muscles | Difficulty in swallowing |
| Unexplained sore throat/fever | Unusual bleeding or bruising |
| Pale skin | Redness or peeling of skin |
| Unusual fatigue | Yellowing of eyes or skin |

# LUNGS

Mucus in the lungs is a chronic inflammatory disease of the lungs. It may result from croup, pneumonia, fibrinous pleurisy, bronchial pneumonia, and irritations from inhaling air pollution. Symptoms are cough, expectoration, and difficult breathing. Enemas have been helpful in cleaning poisons from the body to give it a chance to heal itself. Bronchitis is an infection in the bronchial tubes. Fever can occur. It is also accompanied by back and muscle pain, sore throat and a dry cough. Asthma is a chronic respiratory condition characterized by difficulty in breathing, frequent coughing, and a feeling of suffocation. Attacks can be caused by emotional and physical stress, respiratory infection, air pollution or a change in the temperature. The lungs are one of the elimination organs. Susceptibility to respiratory diseases are increased with air pollution, cigarette smoking, fatigue, chilling, malnutrition and allergic reactions.

## HERBAL COMBINATION NO. 1

*Marshmallow:* heals and soothes lung tissues, eliminates toxins
*Fenugreek:* softens and dissolves hardened mucus, expels phlegm and mucus, kills infections

## HERBAL COMBINATION NO. 2

*Marshmallow:* heals and restores new cell tissues
*Mullein:* has antibiotic properties for upper respiratory system
*Slippery Elm:* helps in inflammation of the mucous membranes, coats and soothes
*Lobelia:* relaxes and clears the air passages of the lungs of viscid material
*Chinese Ephedra:* purges the lungs, cleans and stimulants the bronchial tubes and lungs.
*Passionflower:* relaxing and healing, protects the body from stress for better healing.
*Catnip:* calms the nerves, relaxes spasms and relieves pain, eliminates mucous and increases circulation.

*Senega:* natural expectorant for respiratory problems, increases secretions and circulation.

## HERBAL COMBINATION NO. 3

*Comfrey:* removes mucus from the lungs, healing and soothing tonic

*Marshmallow:* soothes irritated tissues of the lungs, removes difficult phlegm, relaxes the bronchial tubes

*Chickweed:* antiseptic to the blood, soothing to stomach and bowels, cleansing

*Mullein:* calming to irritated nerves, relieves pain, induces relaxed sleep, contains potassium and it is thought that the lack of potassium in the body which causes asthma

## OTHER USES

| | |
|---|---|
| Allergies | Asthma |
| Bronchitis | Coughs |
| Croup | Emphysema |
| Hay Fever | Lung Congestion |
| Mucus | Pneumonia |
| Sinus Problems | Upper Respiratory System |

## SPECIAL DIETARY AIDS

*Vitamin A:* good for healing lung tissue

*Vitamin B-complex:* (especially B12) builds the blood

*Vitamin B6:* deficiency occurs in some asthma patients

*Vitamin C:* fights infection and speeds healing

*Vitamin D:* works with vitamin A to help body withstand diseases

*Vitamin E:* helps guard against air pollution, helps the body to use oxygen more efficiently in lung problems

*Bioflavonoids with Rutin:* works with Vitamin C to strengthen capillaries

*Multi-Vitamin And Mineral (Natural):* for overall body strength

*Folic Acid:* helps strengthen lungs

*Potassium:* found in tomatoes, lettuce, turnips, dandelion greens, celery, egg plant, radishes, fresh string beans, brussel sprouts, kohlrabi, and melons

*Barley Water:* contains hordenine, which relieves bronchial spasms

*Diet, Cleansing:* helps eliminate mucus; during a cleansing diet, germs are burned up or oxidized and eliminated and mucus is dispelled from the lungs

*Garlic:* acts as an antibiotic in killing germs, helps dissolve mucus from the bronchial tubes, lungs and sinus passages

*Honey:* cleans the lungs, soothes coughing spasms

*Juice, Fruit Fasts:* cleans and nourishes the body

*Juice, Grape:* clears the mucus and phlegm from the lungs

*Vinegar And Water:* has a cleansing effect

*Water, Pure:* loss of fluids increases need

*Teas, Herbal:* cleans cells and provides nourishment

*Fresh Pineapple, Berries:* most sour fruits help to dissolve mucus from the lungs

## ORTHODOX PRESCRIBED MEDICATION

### ANTIBIOTICS

Antibiotics like penicillin are often prescribed for respiratory tract infections. Their common side effects include:

| | |
|---|---|
| Hives | Itching |
| Rash | Wheezing |
| Diarrhea | Nausea and vomiting |
| Blood in the urine | Swelling of face and ankles |

### TETRACYCLINE

This is often prescribed for bronchitis and sore throat in children. Its common side effects include:

| | |
|---|---|
| Deformity in developing teeth | Interferes with bone growth |
| Stomach upset | Rash |
| Diarrhea | Sore mouth |

### PREDNISONE AND ISOPROTERENOL

These two medications are widely used for bronchial asthma. Their possible side effects include:

| | |
|---|---|
| Convulsions | Glaucoma |
| Peptic ulcer | Stunted growth in children |

# MENOPAUSE

**M**enopause is that period in a women's life which marks the permanent cessation of menstrual activity. It usually occurs between the ages of 35 to 58. Surgical menopause occurs in almost 30 percent of U.S. women aged 50 to 64. Menopausal symptoms include hot flashes, calcium disturbances, insomnia, diminished interest in sex, irritability, and instability. Poor diet, lack of exercise and emotional stress may increase the symptoms of menopause.

## HERBAL COMBINATION NO. 1

*Black Cohosh:* contains natural estrogen, helps hot flashes, acts as a sedative to contract the uterus

*Licorice:* stimulates adrenal glands, contains estrogen, supplies energy

*False Unicorn:* stimulates reproductive organs, helps in uterine disorders, headaches and depression

*Siberian Ginseng:* stimulates the entire body, nourishes the blood, corrects hormonal imbalance

*Sarsaparilla:* contains progesterone and cortin to help achieve glandular balance

*Squaw Vine:* uterine tonic, helps kidneys to eliminate urine
*Blessed Thistle:* good for menstrual disorders, headaches, tonic

## Other Uses

Hormone Imbalance
Gland Malfunctioning
Morning Sickness
Uterus Problems

Hot Flashes
Menstrual Problems
Sexual Impotency

## Special Dietary Aids

*Vitamin A:* helps in maintaining normal glandular activity
*Vitamin B-complex:* for nerves and iron absorption
*Vitamin B6:* relieves swelling and water retention
*Vitamin C:* helps build resistance to infection
*Rutin:* helps in hemorrhoids, strengthens capillaries
*Vitamin E:* increases production of hormones, promotes the functions of the sexual glands, helps relieve hot flashes
*Vitamin F:* promotes healing and builds tissues
*Multi-Vitamin And Mineral:* take in natural form
*Pantothenic And PABA:* relieves nervous irritability
*Calcium And Phosphorus Balance:* bone meal, calcium can relieve hot flashes
*Iron:* for energy and oxygen
*Magnesium:* works with B-complex to control the nerves
*Potassium:* helps relieve swelling and muscle cramps
*Acidophilus:* can help with vaginitis and cystitis
*Brewer's Yeast:* gives strength to the body, nourishes the cells
*Garlic:* can help in yeast infection
*Kelp:* excellent for anemia

## ORTHODOX PRESCRIBED MEDICATION

### ESTROGEN

Estrogen therapy is essentially a hormone-replacement therapy. Its common side effects are:

Blood clots

Pains in chest, groins, and legs

Speech, slurred, sudden

Vision changes

Cramps of lower stomach

Nausea

Breast, lumps

Headache, severe, sudden

Loss of coordination

Shortness of breath

Loss of appetite

Swelling of ankles and feet

# MIGRAINE HEADACHES

**M**igraine headaches are a type of headache due to the alternating constriction or dilation of the blood vessels in the brain. The exact cause is unknown, but emotional stress is thought to play a large role. The symptoms include intense pain, nausea, vomiting, and visual problems.

## HERBAL COMBINATION NO. 1

*Fenugreek:* kills infection, strong antiseptic

*Thyme:* antiseptic and healing powers, cleans stomach

## OTHER USES

Bronchitis

Fevers

Heartburn

Sinus Congestion

Digestion

Headache

Mucus

Worms

## SPECIAL DIETARY AIDS

*Vitamin B-complex:* general nutrition, stimulant, utilizes energy in brain and nervous tissues

*Vitamin C:* if used daily will help protect from stress

*Calcium:* calms nerves, needed in stressful times

*Lecithin:* helps control the nerves

*Multi-Mineral:* strengthens the system

*Niacin:* prevents nervous disorders, promotes good physical and mental health

*Rutin:* needed for healthy capillaries

*Water, Pure:* cleans the system

*Brewer's Yeast:* contains complete protein and B-complex, very helpful in migraine headaches

*Carrot And Celery Juice:* relieves migraine headaches

*Sprouts:* high in chlorophyll which is the life blood of plants, and is similar to human blood

*Vinegar:* (apple cider) with honey in water has been said to relieve migraine headaches

## ORTHODOX PRESCRIBED MEDICATION

### INDERAL

Inderal has become popular for migraine headaches. In older persons (over sixty), Inderal seems to be eliminated from the body more slowly, so these people are more susceptible to side effects. Its possible side effects include:

| | |
|---|---|
| Fatigue | Weakness |
| Light: headedness | Stomach upset |
| Diarrhea | Breathing, (difficult) |

### METHYSERIDGE

This is a widely claimed cure for migraines. Its side effects include:

Ankles, swollen
Indigestion
Weight increase

Cramps in calves of legs
Hair (falling out)

# NERVOUS DISORDERS

Nervous disorders are manifested by the instability of nerve action, excitability, the state of restlessness, mental or physical or both. The nervous system is vital to life. The nervous system transmits all sensory input, sound, sight, taste, smell and touch to the brain and controls the workings of the organs. It helps maintain the temperature of the body and blood pressure. Causes of disorders can include lack of proper nutrition and organic disorders, overwork, worry, noisy surroundings and physical problems. Exercise, including breathing exercises (one nostril at a time), helps relieve many nervous disorders.

## HERBAL COMBINATION NO. 1

*Black Cohosh:* contains alkaloid properties for nerves

*Capsicum:* stimulating to distribute other herbs to needed parts of the body

*Valerian:* pain reliever, relaxing for nervous tension

*Ginger:* helps hold together all herbs, helps relaxant herbs work more effectively

*White Willow:* natural pain reliever, sedative for the nerves, healing for the stomach and intestines.

*Devil's Claw:* blood cleanser, anti-inflammatory properties, pain reliever.

*Hops:* its sedative properties make an excellent relaxant, contains B vitamins for nerves

*Wood Betony:* useful when used with other herbs

# HERBAL COMBINATION NO. 2

*Black Cohosh:* soothing effect on the nervous system, lowers blood pressure

*Capsicum:* stimulates other herbs to be more effective, increases blood circulation, helps eliminates toxic wastes

*Valerian:* sedative effect on the entire system, remedy for nervous disorders

*Lady's Slipper:* tonic for exhausted nervous system, calming to body and mind

*Passionflower:* relaxes the nerves, good for strengthening the nervous system, has natural pain reliever properties

*Skullcap:* controls nervous irritations, good for insomnia due to overactive mind

*Hops:* general tonic, sleep inducer, sedative to the nervous system

*Wood Betony:* cleans impurities from blood, effective sedative

## OTHER USES

| | |
|---|---|
| Anxiety | Convulsions |
| Headaches | Hyperactivity |
| Hysteria | Insomnia |
| Nervous Breakdown | Relaxant |

## SPECIAL DIETARY AIDS

*Vitamin A:* works with vitamins D and E to fight infections and promote growth repair of body tissues.

*B-Vitamins:* necessary for normal functioning of the nervous system

*Vitamin B1:* important to a healthy nervous system and affects mental attitude

*Vitamin B3:* helps relieve depression

*Vitamin B12:* necessary for healthy nerves and brain, prevents nervous disorders

*Vitamin B6:* soothing effect on nerves, prevents nervous disorders

*Vitamin C:* works with vitamin D in the regulation of calcium metabolism, promotes health in the system, lack of vitamin C causes irritability

*Calcium:* relaxing and calming to the nerves, manganese is necessary for proper absorption

*Vitamin D:* also a nerve vitamin, helps to relax

*Iron:* promotes a sense of well-being, increases energy and vitality

*Lysine (Amino Acid):* lack causes irritability

*Magnesium:* feeds the nerves, helps emotional disturbances

*Pantothenic Acid:* strengthens to withstand stress

*Potassium:* strengthens the nervous system

*Tyrosine (Amino Acid):* controls depression, along with B6 and niacin

*Apples:* health tonic and regulates the bowels, apples are said to prevent emotional upsets, tension and headaches

*Artichokes:* cleans the kidneys, helps with poor digestion

*Blackstrap Molasses:* rich in iron, gives the body energy

*Bran:* contains natural amino acids, necessary for healthy body, keeps the colon clean

*Brewer's Yeast:* supplies live protein and B vitamins

*Brussels Sprouts:* tonic food, good for catarrh build up

*Cauliflower:* purifies the blood, rich in minerals

*Fruit:* papaya, guava, acerola, gives nourishment to the body, aids digestion, cleans the digestive tract

*Lettuce:* calming to the nerves

*Teas:* Fenugreek and Chamomile teas are excellent for many of the body's systems

*Vegetables, Raw Juices:* carrot, beet and cabbage, cleansing and nourishing to the body

*Wheat Germ:* excellent source of the B-complex vitamins

*Whole Grains:* buckwheat, barley, millet

## ORTHODOX PRESCRIBED MEDICATION

### VALIUM

Valium is prescribed for nervous tension. Its common side effects include:

| | |
|---|---|
| Clumsiness | Unsteadiness |
| Dizziness | Drowsiness |
| Blurred vision | Constipation |
| Diarrhea | Headache |
| Heartburn | Withdrawal symptoms |
| Nausea | Slurred speech |
| Stomach pains | Unusual fatigue |

# PANCREAS AND DIABETES

The pancreas gland performs two important functions . It is necessary to produce the pancreatic acid juice which is used to help digestion, and it also produces insulin. Pancreatitis symptoms can be acid indigestion, nausea, pain and gas. The weakness for diabetes can be inherited, so it is important to strengthen the pancreas gland, digestive system and the colon.

## HERBAL COMBINATION NO. 1

*Goldenseal:* natural insulin, regulates sugar in the blood, feeds glands, builds resistance to diseases

*Juniper Berries:* high in natural insulin, helps restore function of the pancreas

*Uva Ursi:* helps regulate sugar levels, helps alleviate pancreas disorders

*Mullein:* antibiotic properties, nourishes body strength, calms nerves

*Yarrow:* blood cleanser, dilates the pores, producing sweating, removes congestion

*Garlic:* stimulates cell growth and activity, rejuvenates body functions

*Capsicum:* helps heal pancreas, increases and regulates circulation, nourishes

*Dandelion:* increases activity of the pancreas, clears obstructions, purifies the blood, tonic

*Marshmallow:* healing to the system, removes phlegm, high in vitamin A and minerals

*Licorice:* increases strength of other herbs, supplies energy to system

*Nettle:* diuretic, astringent,and antibiotic properties, high in iron, silicon, potassium, and is rich in vitamin A and C. Increases circulation and is healing for the intestinal system.

*White Oak:* strengthens the glands, prevents bleeding, contains healing and nourishing properties. Natural diuretic to clean the urinary tract.

## Herbal Combination No. 2

*Cedar Berries:* antiseptic, healing and nourishing for the pancreas, dissolves toxins, increases the flow of urine, cleans the blood.

*Burdock:* great blood cleanser, prevents accumulation of toxins in the body, rich in inulin which is nourishing and healing for the pancreas, helps balance hormones.

*Horseradish:* antibiotic properties to dissolve and eliminate toxins, prevents infections.

*Siberian Ginseng:* strengthens the entire body, increases circulation and mental alertness. Cleans the blood, improves glandular function.

## OTHER USES

| | |
|---|---|
| Blood Sugar Problems | Gallbladder |
| Hyperglycemia | Glucose Intolerance |
| Glycosuria | Kidney |
| Liver | Spleen |

## SPECIAL DIETARY AIDS

*Essential Fatty Acids:* The most prominent EFAs include Flaxseed, Borage, Black Currant, Evening Primrose, and Fish Oils. They nourish and feed the glands.

*Digestive Enzymes:* necessary to strengthen the pancreas, and clean the undigested protein from the blood and cells.

*Free-Form Amino Acids:* essential for healing the glands and nourish and strengthen the body.

*Blue-green Algae and Chlorophyll:* supplies nutrients, and cleans the blood and glands. Rebuilds damaged pancreas.

*Vitamin A:* assists in maintaining normal glandular activity

*Vitamin B-complex:* general nutritional stimulant

*Vitamin C:* promotes glandular activity, helps infections

*Vitamin E:* reduces uric acid, increases production of hormones

*Calcium:* calms nerves, builds blood, promotes enzyme stimulation

*Magnesium:* stimulates the glands, alkalizes the system

*Manganese:* essential element, acts as an activator for enzymes

*Niacin:* promotes growth by stimulating metabolic processes

*Potassium:* increases glandular secretions

*Zinc:* aids entire hormonal system and all the glands

*Fruits, Raw, Fresh:* cleans the intestines, nourishes

*Molasses:* rich in iron

*Nuts:* contains protein needed for cells

*Seeds, Pumpkin:* cleansing and nourishing to the body, helps carry nourishment to various parts of the body

*Vegetables, Green Leafy:* supplies live enzymes

*Raw Food:* stimulates the pancreas to increase insulin production
*Protein:* (such as cottage cheese, yogurt, kefir, nuts and seeds, and
avocado), is necessary for all the cells of the body

## ORTHODOX PRESCRIBED MEDICATION

### INSULIN

Insulin belongs to the group of medicines called hormones. If the body does not make enough insulin to meet its needs, a condition known as diabetes mellitus (sugar diabetes) may develop. Eating the right foods along with proper exercise plus insulin helps keep health in balance. Insulin is made from beef or pork sources, and many insulin preparations contain mixtures of both. Insulin must be injected under the skin, because when taken by mouth, it is destroyed by stomach acid. Insulin reaction may occur and the symptoms are:

| | |
|---|---|
| Anxiety | Chills |
| Cold sweats | Cool pale skin |
| Drowsiness | Excessive hunger |
| Headache | Nausea |
| Nervousness | Rapid pulse |
| Shakiness | Unusual fatigue or weakness |

# PAIN

A disturbed sensation where a person suffers discomfort or distress due to provocation of sensory nerves. Pain is a symptom, and the reason for the pain is the important thing to seek. There could be many reasons for pain in the system. It could cause emotional stress with lack of sleep. Therefore, it is important to find a natural relief for pain. An herbal calcium formula will help rebuild the nervous system so the body can relieve pain naturally. It should contain horsetail and oatstraw. Herbal nervine formulas will strengthen the nervous system and they should contain some of the following: hops, skullcap, passionflower, valerian, white willow, or chamomile.

## HERBAL COMBINATION NO. 1

*White Willow:* natural pain reliever, contains antiseptic properties and is cleansing and healing.
*Valerian:* nerve tonic, relieves headache pain
*Wild Lettuce:* helps after-birth pains, general pain reliever
*Capsicum:* stimulant, relaxant

## OTHER USES

| | |
|---|---|
| After: birth pain | Cramps |
| Headache | Relaxant |
| Toothache | |

## SPECIAL DIETARY AIDS

*Vitamin B-complex:* especially B1, B3, B6, and B12, calming to the nerves
*Vitamin A:* lubricates all membranes to help keep them clean and free from virus infections
*Vitamin C:* detoxifies germs in body
*Vitamin D:* relaxes nerves and helps calcium to absorb
*Vitamin E:* dilates capillary blood vessels to lessen pain
*Calcium:* helps in menstrual pain, calms nerves
*Folic Acid:* needed under stress and disease
*Magnesium:* helps the nervous system, it promotes sleep
*Pantothenic Acid:* helps the body to withstand stress
*Fruit, Juices:* assimilates quickly into the blood stream
*Vegetables, Fresh, Juices:* cleans and nourishes the body
*Wild Yam:* has been used for many kinds of pain

## ORTHODOX PRESCRIBED MEDICATION

### ASPIRIN

Aspirin and related products are often used for treating pain, fever and inflammation. Their side effects include:

| | |
|---|---|
| Stomach irritation | Brain hemorrhage |
| Birth defects | Arteriosclerosis |
| Ringing in the ears | Nausea |
| Bleeding stomach | Allergic reaction |
| Ulcers, ulcer damage | |

# PARASITES (WORMS)

A parasite is an organism that lives within, upon, or at the expense of another organism, known as the host, without contributing to the survival of the host. Parasites are said to affect a large percentage of our population, causing many symptoms often blamed on other conditions such as pneumonia, jaundice or periodontitis. Symptoms can include diarrhea, hunger pain, appetite loss, weight loss and anemia. Tapeworms can be contracted from eating insufficiently cooked meats; especially beef, pork, and fish.

## HERBAL COMBINATION NO. 1

*Pumpkin Seeds:* expels tapeworms efficiently, nutritious
*Violet:* contains properties that will reach places only the blood and lymphatic fluids penetrate
*Black Walnut:* oxygenates the blood to kill parasites and worms, burns up toxins and fatty deposits.
*Chamomile:* soothing and relaxing so the body can heal itself, cleans and nourishes

*Marshmallow:* soothing and healing for the mucous membranes, rich in vitamin A, and high contents of calcium and zinc.

*Cascara Sagrada:* safe laxative and cleanser, stimulating effect on the colon

*Mullein:* calming effect on all inflamed and irritated nerves, good for bleeding bowels

*Slippery Elm:* soothes and disperses inflammation, draws out impurities, heals all parts of the body

*Elecampane:* expels worms with its antiseptic properties, healing and nourishing, tonic and expectorant properties.

*Spearmint:* soothing and calming to the intestinal tract, relieves pain and muscle spasms, increases circulation to speed healing.

*Turmeric:* improves digestion, and liver function, may be effective for destroying amoebae which can cause dysentery.

*Garlic:* natural antibiotic, kills bacteria, parasites and worms, cleans and strengthens the blood vessels.

*Ginger:* cleansing and healing properties for the intestinal tract, settles stomach, and has pain relieving properties.

*Clove:* good for pain, nausea and vomiting, increases circulation to promote healing.

## Other Uses

| | |
|---|---|
| Bowel (Cleans) | Cancer |
| Prostate | Tumors |

## Special Dietary Aids

*Vitamin A:* improves resistance to infections in the gastrointestinal tract

*Vitamin B-complex:* builds blood, tones muscles, acts as a general nutrition stimulant

*Vitamin B6:* promotes appetite, digestion, assimilation and elimination

*Vitamin B12:* improves blood supply, promotes growth, prevents nervous disorders

*Vitamin C:* detoxifies the body and strengthens the body

*Vitamin D:* necessary for good body form and health

*Vitamin K:* aids in blood coagulation and controls consistency

*Calcium:* promotes enzyme stimulation, calms nerves, used as a painkiller

*Iron:* increases energy and vitality, alkalizes the system

*Fruits, Fresh, Raw:* promotes healthy body with live enzymes

*Garlic:* antibiotic, helps destroy parasites

*Vegetables, Fresh, Raw:* promotes healthy body with live enzymes A clean colon will help eliminate the breeding place for parasites. Whole wheat bread, instead of white; honey, instead of white sugar; natural vitamins and minerals, instead of those made in a laboratory, should be used.

## Orthodox Prescribed Medication

### Pyrvinium (Povan)

This is used for pinworm infestations. This medicine is a dye and will cause the stools to be red. It may also stain the teeth. Its possible side effects are:

Nausea, vomiting                    Skin rash
Diarrhea                            Dizziness
Unusual sensitivity to sunlight     Stomach cramps

# PRENATAL CARE

There are a lot of changes in a pregnant woman, both mental and physical. The blood supply increases, there can be nausea, and the need for sleep increases. The nutritional needs of the mother increase, and the condition of the child as well as the mother could be improved by dietary supplementation. One way to prepare for the delivery of the child is with the use of herbs. They have been found to help strengthen the uterus for safe and easy delivery.

## HERBAL COMBINATION NO. 1

*Black Cohosh:* controls hemorrhaging, nervousness and delivery pains; reduces high blood pressure

*Squaw Vine:* useful for urinary and vaginal infections, helps facilitate delivery, strengthens uterus in childbirth

*Dong Quai:* natural relaxer and strengthener of the uterus, prevents bleeding, cleans blood, nourishes the glands, relaxes muscles for easier childbirth.

*Butcher's Broom:* improves circulation and prevents post-operative thrombosis, varicose veins, and hemorrhoids which are common with pregnancy.

*Red Raspberry:* strengthens uterus, relieves pain, aids in easy labor

## OTHER USES

| | |
|---|---|
| Child Birth | Menstrual Cramps |
| Uterus (Strengthens) | Delivery |

## SPECIAL DIETARY AIDS

*Vitamin B-complex:* especially B6, soothes the nerves, increases relaxation, restores sleep, prevents morning sickness and nausea in pregnancy

*Vitamin C:* kills infections, promotes formation of healthy teeth, strengthens blood vessels, builds resistance to infections

*Vitamin D:* regulates mineral metabolism of bones, teeth and nails

*Vitamin K:* to help blood coagulation and to prevent hemorrhages in delivery

*Bioflavonoids:* to strengthen blood vessels

*Calcium:* high amounts needed for bones teeth

*Iron:* enriches blood, feeds tissues, nourishes the glands

*Thiamine:* in late pregnancy, builds the blood, tones muscles, nutritional stimulant, feeds nerves

*Fruits, Fresh:* gives strength and nourishment to the body

*Protein:* gives daily nourishment of the cells (milk, yogurt, whole grains, nuts, beans, lentils, eggs, cheese and fish)

*Vegetables, Fresh:* gives necessary vitamins and minerals to the body

# PROSTATE

Prostatitis is an inflammation of the male sex gland, the prostate. Herbs can play an important role to a healthy prostate, bladder and kidney function. It can help in keeping these free from infection. Herbs help in the relief of chronic irritations of the bladder. Eating correct food and getting sufficient exercise in the fresh air also helps.

## HERBAL COMBINATION NO. 1

*Black Cohosh:* stimulates secretions of the liver, kidneys and Iymph glands, expels mucus

*Licorice:* removes excess fluid from the body, supplies energy, acts as a natural cortisone

*Kelp:* promotes glandular health, relieves inflammation and reduces pain in glands

*Gotu Kola:* natural diuretic, defends body against toxins, helps with hormone balance

*Goldenseal:* antibiotic and antiseptic to stop infection, eliminates toxins from bladder

*Capsicum:* stimulating, reduces glandular swellings, distributes other herbs

*Ginger:* helps remove excess waste from system, enhances effectiveness of other herbs, stimulates

*Dong Quai:* increases circulation for better healing, prevents bleeding, strengthens and nourishes the glands.

## HERBAL COMBINATION NO. 2

*Pygeum:* used in Europe and Africa successfully for prostate problems. Reduces swelling and inflammation, dissolves deposits that can block urination.

*Saw Palmetto:* cleans and feeds the glands, contains natural antibiotic properties to help in infections and enlarged prostate.

*Stinging Nettle:* rich in minerals, which helps when acids are irritating the body, heals, eliminates excess water, and nourishes the glands.

*Gotu Kola:* blood cleanser, stimulates mental and physical energy, mental alertness, considered a brain and nervous system nutrient.

*Zinc:* necessary for prostate health, essential for cell division, repair and growth, very healing for wounds and infections.

## OTHER USES

| | |
|---|---|
| Bladder | Hormone Regulator |
| Kidneys | Liver |
| Spleen | Urinary Tract |

## SPECIAL DIETARY AIDS

*Vitamin A:* helps in tension, irritability; helps infections

*Vitamin B-complex:* especially B6, helps in hormone balance

*Vitamin C:* helps resist infection

*Vitamin E:* essential for reproduction, stimulates male hormone

*Vitamin F:* aids in prostate gland problems

*Zinc:* helps absorb B vitamin stimulates prostate

*Calcium:* helps minerals to absorb

*Magnesium:* necessary for calcium and vitamin C metabolism

*Almonds And Sesame Seeds:* high in calcium and potassium, valuable for nourishing the cells

*Artichokes:* cleanses the prostate and urinary tract

*Asparagus:* natural diuretic

*Bee Pollen:* stimulates male potency, heals prostate troubles

*Grains:* contains quality proteins and the B-complex vitamin

*Pumpkin Seeds:* healing and nourishing to the prostate and urinary tract

*Raw Fruits and Vegetables:* provides enzymes necessary for healthy system

*Sunflower Seeds:* high in protein and enzymes

*Water:* drink lots of pure water to clean the system

*Watercress and Parsley:* both of these are natural diuretic

## ORTHODOX PRESCRIBED MEDICATION

### NALIDIXIC ACID

This is commonly prescribed for prostate infection. Its common side effects include:

| | |
|---|---|
| Blurred or decreased vision | Double vision |
| Change in color vision | Diarrhea |
| Itching | Nausea |
| Sensitivity to bright lights | Halos around lights |
| Rash | Vomiting |
| Dizziness | Drowsiness |
| Dark urine | Pale skin |
| Pale stools | Severe stomach pain |
| Unusual bleeding | Unexplained sore throat/fever |
| Unusual fatigue or weakness | Yellowing of eyes or skin |

# REDUCING WEIGHT

*L*osing weight is a matter of curbing the amount of food calories eaten, and increasing daily activities. There is no easy road to reducing. The American public should stop hoping for an easy way to lose weight. The only hope is to stop believing that there is one, and start changing to thin eating habits. It has taken years to accumulate excess weight and it will take months to lose. Herbs can help the body adjust as well as supply vitamins and minerals. This combination acts as a general body cleanser, regulates metabolism, dissolves fat in the body, helps eliminate craving for food, stimulates glandular secretions, reduces water retention, boosts energy and helps in constipation.

## HERBAL COMBINATION NO. 1

*Chickweed:* dissolves fat in blood vessels, potassium content helps eliminate craving for food

*Licorice:* gives energy boost, counteracts stress, helps balance other herbs

*Safflower:* helps produce more adrenaline, natural insulin, digestive aid

*Cascara Sagrada:* promotes natural peristaltic action to clean and restore natural tone to the colon. Increases the flow of bile to improve liver and gallbladder function, good for chronic constipation.

*Parthenium:* natural blood cleanser, eliminates water retention, soothing and healing to the colon.

*Black Walnut:* balances sugar levels, burns excess toxins and fatty materials

*Gotu Kola:* feeds the brain, energizes cells of the brain

*Hawthorn:* strengthens heart, helps circulation, good for nerves and stress

*Papaya:* calms nervous stomach, and aids digestion

*Fennel:* cleans mucous membranes of intestinal tract, and removes waste from body

*Dandelion:* strengthens liver, helps in water retention and destroys acids

## OTHER USES

| | |
|---|---|
| Energy | Constipation |
| Cleanser | Water Retention |

## SPECIAL DIETARY AIDS

*Essential Fatty Acids:* necessary for the glands to produce the hormones and enzymes to balance the body to lose and maintain ideal weight.

*Digestive Enzymes:* essential to digest and assimilate food properly to prevent overeating. Also prevents undigested food from causing congestion in the blood and organs.

*Vitamin B-complex:* especially B6 and B12, necessary for normal metabolism of nerve tissue and is involved in protein, fat and carbohydrate metabolism

*Vitamin C:* increases alertness, promotes health

*Vitamin E:* promotes circulation, reduces uric acid

*Vitamin F:* improves heart action

*Phenylalanine (Natural Amino Acid):* has an effect on the thyroid to help weight control, depresses the appetite

*Calcium:* calms the nerves, promotes sleep, builds the blood, assists

*Lecithin:* helps break up the fatty material in body, distributes body weight, maintains healthy nervous system.

*Magnesium:* stimulate the glands, creates good disposition

*Protein (Vegetable):* such as in grains, seeds and nuts

*Brewer's Yeast:* strengthens the body and gives energy

*Kelp:* helps regulate thyroid for metabolism

*Pineapple:* aid to digestion to help rid the body of excess weight
*Watercress:* rich in minerals and vitamins and chlorophyll
*Wheat Germ:* contains vitamin B-complex protein

## ORTHODOX PRESCRIBED MEDICATION

### DEXEDRINE

Dexedrine is usually prescribed for short-term adjunct to caloric restriction. It could also be habit-forming. Its common side effects include:

| | |
|---|---|
| False sense of well-being | Irritability |
| Nervousness | Restlessness |

# SEX REJUVENATION

This combination has been used for male hormone problems such as impotence. The main impact on the male hormone testosterone is on the emotions. If production were to cease, it would produce irritable, fretful, and sleepless feelings. Memory would begin to fail, and some men feel the hot flashes that women often have at menopause. This formula will help to improve the hormone balance, build the reproductive glands, help prostate function, reduce frigidity, infertility, hot flashes, impotence, fatigue and other menopausal problems.

## HERBAL COMBINATION NO. 1

*Siberian Ginseng:* antistress, benefits heart and circulation, stimulates body energy, contains male hormone, testosterone, helps correct impotence
*Saw Palmetto:* effective hormone herb useful on reproductive glands, and is said to increase the size of small breasts

*Gotu Kola:* rebuilds energy reserve, helps in nervous disorders, strengthens heart, brain and nerves, helps with hormone balance

*Damiana:* helps balance female hormones, hot flashes, stimulating to the system, increases sperm count in the male and strengthens the egg in the female, helps in sexual impotence

*Sarsaparilla:* contains progesterone for glandular balance, stimulates circulation, contains male hormone, testosterone

*Parthenium:* cleans blood and liver to help eliminate infections, increases blood flow, soothing and healing.

*Horsetail:* rich in silicon to increase absorption of calcium, increases circulation, natural diuretic, and will shrink inflamed tissues.

*Garlic:* natural antibiotic, reduces blood pressure, stimulates cell growth

*Capsicum:* stimulates other herbs to the location where they are needed, wards off disease, increases blood circulation

*Chickweed:* dissolves plaque out of blood vessels, contains antiseptic properties

## OTHER USES

| | |
|---|---|
| Frigidity | Hot Flashes |
| Menopause | Sexual Stimulant |

## SPECIAL DIETARY AIDS

*Vitamin A:* lessens premenstrual tension and irritability

*Vitamin B-complex:* especially B6, helps in hormonal and sugar balance

*Vitamin C and Bioflavonoids:* increases capillary strength

*Vitamin D:* relaxes nerves

*Vitamin E:* male hormone energizer which helps build up the male sex glands for youthful hormone balance

*Vitamin F:* alleviates female problems

*Calcium And Magnesium:* helps correct hormone rhythm, nerve foods

*Dolomite And Bone Meal:* contains calcium so necessary for overall healthy feeling

*Iron:* enriches blood

*Manganese Pantothenic Acid and PABA:* relieves nervous irritability

*Zinc:* stimulates prostate glands

*Protein (Not Red Meat):* grains, nuts and seeds, wheat germ, polished rice

*Seeds, Sunflower and Pumpkin:* stimulates male potency and heals prostate problems

*Tea, Fenugreek:* soothing on the urinary tract, keeping it free from mucus and pus

*Tea, Parsley:* relieves bladder irritations, high in vitamin A, has a moisturizing effect on mucous lining of prostate gland

*Vegetables, Fresh:* live enzymes, nourishment

## ORTHODOX PRESCRIBED MEDICATION

### ANDROID

Android is prescribed for impotence. Its possible side effects include:

| | |
|---|---|
| Skin rash | Shock |
| Deficient sperm count | Abnormal mammaries in male |

# SKIN, HAIR AND NAILS

The skin is the largest eliminative organ of the body. If it is functioning properly, it eliminates as much as the kidneys and the lungs. Sun and fresh air are important to the skin. Olive oil or aloe vera are good for sunbathing, for they do not plug the pores. The use of a loofah or sponge is useful when bathing to stimulate and tone the skin and remove dead skin from the body. The following herbal combination is also useful for general hair and nail care.

## HERBAL COMBINATION NO. 1

*Dulse:* high in iodine, high in minerals and vitamins needed for the skin, hair and nails

*Horsetail:* helps prevent falling hair and strengthens nails and tones the skin, high in minerals

*Sage:* stimulates hair growth, an astringent and acts as a scalp tonic

*Rosemary:* strengthens eye sight, stimulates the skin and strengthens the hair

## SPECIAL DIETARY AIDS

*Essential Fatty Acids:* the skin, hair and nails needs natural oils to soften and prevent brittle nails, to keep the hair healthy and shinny, and the skin from becoming dry and wrinkled. Flaxseed, Borage, Black Currant, Evening Primrose and Fish Oils are the primary EFAs.

*Free-Form Amino Acids:* essential for healthy skin, hair and nails, which are mostly made of protein and need to be nourished.

*Vitamin A:* promotes healthy skin

*Vitamin B-complex:* especially B2 (promotes healthier skin) and B6 (helps prevent acne)

*Vitamin D:* necessary for good body form

*Vitamin E:* good for liver spots

*Calcium:* promotes skin healing

*Zinc:* helps in tissue respiration

*Blackstrap Molasses:* provides iron for rich blood

*Brewer's Yeast:* contains protein and B vitamins

*Diet:* a cleansing diet is beneficial for cleaning the blood to promote healthy skin

*Fruits, Fresh, Raw:* cleans the blood to help keep the skin clear and healthy looking

*Garlic:* the oil heals blisters, boils can be helped with oil and garlic, kills staphylococci germs in boils, heals running sores

*Grains, Whole:* brown rice and millet, gives the body necessary protein for healthy skin

*Honey:* good for sting bites

*Lecithin:* helps in the structural support of all cells, especially the nerves and brain

*Lemon Juice:* helps skin conditions

*Sprouts:* promotes healthy skin with enzyme, vitamins and mineral content

*Seeds, Sunflower:* protein, natural food, helps dry skin

*Vegetables, Fresh, Raw:* nourishes the blood for healthy skin and body

*Wheat Germ Oil:* good for insect stings and bites Avoid excess fat and sweets and any products with white flour and sugar

# THYROID

The chief function of the thyroid gland is to regulate the rate of metabolism. Goiter may be caused by a lack of iodine in the diet, inflammation of the thyroid gland due to infection or under or over production of hormones by the thyroid gland.

## HERBAL COMBINATION NO. 1

*Irish Moss:* purifies and strengthens the cellular structure and vital fluids of the system

*Kelp:* promotes glandular health, highest natural source of iodine, rich in minerals, strengthens tissues in the brain and heart

*Black Walnut:* helps to balance sugar levels, natural source of iodine, burns up excess toxins

*Parsley:* increases resistance to infection and diseases, high in potassium, regulates the fluids, tonic to urinary system

*Watercress:* acts as a tonic for regulating metabolism, blood purifier

*Sarsaparilla:* stimulates the metabolic rate, valuable in glandular balance

*Iceland Moss:* nutrient, tonic, regulates gastric acid

## HERBAL COMBINATION NO. 2

*Kelp:* promotes glandular health, helps control metabolism, high in minerals, cleans colon

*Irish Moss:* purifies and strengthens cellular structure, iodine helps glandular system

*Parsley:* tonic effect to the whole system, increases resistance to disease, high in minerals for healthy metabolism

*Capsicum:* stimulates blood circulation, helps other herbs to be more effective

## HERBAL COMBINATION NO. 3

*Kelp:* rich in natural iodine, essential for thyroid health. Helps speed metabolism to burn excess calories, cleans the veins, strengthens the glands, brain and nerves.

*Irish Moss:* supplies nutrients to sustain glandular health. Soothing, healing and nourishing.

*Parsley:* natural diuretic, rich in vitamins and minerals clean the blood and veins, nourishes the glands

*Hops:* sedative properties help the to relax, where healing is more effective. Strengthens the nervous system.

*Capsicum:* stimulating to increase circulation for better glandular health. Increases effectiveness of other herbs in the combination.

*Zinc:* main healing mineral for proper digestion of proteins, carbohydrates, and essential for proper action of insulin for the pancreas.

*Manganese:* essential for proper function of glands, especially the pituitary, nourishing for the brain, and nerves.

*Glutamine:* an amino acid that help in sugar and alcohol cravings, stimulates mental alertness, detoxifies ammonia from the brain, and helps in behavioral problems.

*Proline:* and amino acid essential for collagen formation, healing for wounds and necessary for healthy tissues.

*Histidine:* an essential amino acid for nerve health, controls the mucous level of the digestive and respiratory system. Helps in controlling stress.

## OTHER USES

| | |
|---|---|
| Energy | Epilepsy |
| Fatigue | Glands |
| Goiter | Hormones |

## SPECIAL DIETARY AIDS

*Vitamin A:* assists in sustaining normal glandular activity

*Vitamin B-complex:* prime source of predigested protein, boosts the thyroid for energy

*Vitamin B6:* protects against stress, aids in formation of antibodies

*Vitamin C:* neutralizes infections, helps promote healthy glandular function

*Vitamin E:* increases production of hormones, improves circulation

*Calcium:* assists all metabolic functions to perform efficiently, promotes enzyme stimulation

*Iodine:* aids in the development and functioning of the thyroid gland and produces the hormone thyroxine, regulates the body's production of energy

*Zinc:* boosts the thyroid for energy

*Brewer's Yeast:* contains nucleic acids and oil

*Eggs, Raw, Fertile:* rich in protein, contains all the amino acids to combine with enzymes to build strong bodies

*Exercise:* daily exercise to circulate the blood which helps the thyroid

*Fruit, Raw, Fresh:* easily assimilated enzyme that contains predigested levulose. The system instantly absorbs levulose to give the body energy and vigor.

*Seeds, Pumpkin:* contains protein, unsaturated fatty acids and minerals which unite with enzymes for a healthy hormonal function

*Seeds, Sunflower:* high in proteins and vitamins and minerals, packed full of the sun

*Sprouts:* live enzymes, easily assimilated, high in vitamins and amino acids, rich in chlorophyll, similar to human blood

*Yogurt:* richest source of enzymes, helps in assimilation of calcium, aids in the manufacture of B-complex, prime source of predigested protein

## ORTHODOX PRESCRIBED MEDICATION

### METHIMAZOLE

This is an antithyroid agent. They are used to treat conditions in which the thyroid gland produces too much thyroid hormone and also before thyroid surgery. Its possible side effects include:

| | |
|---|---|
| Itching | Dizziness |
| Joint pain | Loss of taste |
| Nausea and vomiting | Numbness |
| Tingling of fingers | Skin rash |
| Stomach pain | |

# ULCERS

*U*lcers are open sores or lesions of the skin or mucous membranes of the body, with loss of substance, sometimes accompanied by formation of pus. Some nutritionists call stomach and gastric ulcers a deficiency disease caused by unhealthy tissue as a result of eating incompatible combinations of food leaving fermentation and putrefaction as the end product. Ulcers are seen by many doctors to be caused by bacteria in the digestive system called *Helicobacter pylori.* There are some natural treatments that are effective. Eliminate fried foods, sodium chloride, strong spices, animal fats, alcohol, caffeine and carbonated drinks. Severe nervous and mental stress can cause ulcers. It is important to be able to relax and rest and free the mind of problems and stressful situations.

## HERBAL COMBINATION NO. 1

*Capsicum:* stimulant, hemorrhages, internal disinfectant, high in vitamins and minerals

*Goldenseal:* stops infection, internal bleeding, eliminates toxins from the stomach

*Myrrh Gum:* antiseptic, strengthens digestive system, aids inflammation to speed healing

## OTHER USES

| | |
|---|---|
| Bad Breath | Canker Sores |
| Colitis | Colon |
| Diverticulitis | Dysentery |
| Heartburn | Indigestion |
| Stomach Ulcer | |

## SPECIAL DIETARY AIDS

*Vitamin A:* large amounts at first complaint heals tissues that line the sores

*Vitamin B-complex:* especially B2 and B12, improves the body health and strengthens the nerves

*Vitamin C and Bioflavonoids:* large amounts will help heal ulcers

*Vitamins E and A:* vitamin E helps heal scar tissue

*Vitamin K:* helps in blood clotting

*Iron:* builds rich blood, gives energy to the body

*Raw Cabbage and Potato Juice:* contains vitamin P which helps ulcers heal

*Yogurt:* friendly stomach bacteria, prime source of predigested protein. Eliminate white sugar products and red meat.

*Digestive Enzymes:* very beneficial to digest nutrients as well as break up undigested protein that stay in the stomach because of leaky gut syndrome. Used between meals will help some get into the blood stream and be eliminated.

*Hydrochloric Acid:* essential to break up protein so that it can be digested properly. It will also destroy bacteria, worms and parasites that irritate the intestinal lining.

## ORTHODOX PRESCRIBED MEDICATION

### CIMETIDINE (TAGAMET)

This is often prescribed in treating certain types of ulcers and other gastrointestinal disorders. Its common side effects include:

| | |
|---|---|
| Dizziness | Diarrhea |
| Headaches | Muscle cramps |
| Skin rash | Swelling of breasts |
| Breast soreness | |

# SECTION 5

## *What We Eat*

# Diet/Nutritional Therapies

## CLEANSING AND FASTING

A cleansing diet is good during colds, flu or illness. The body has the ability to rid itself of toxins if it is given the chance. Toxins are expelled through the skin, which needs to be kept clean and scrubbed, and through the nose, mouth, colon and stomach. The purpose of cleansing the body is to eliminate excessive mucus and toxins. The first step is to stay away from white sugar products, white flour products, animal protein and salt.

The benefits of a cleansing fast are many. It dissolves toxins and mucus in the body, it cleanses the kidneys and the digestive system, purifies the glands and the cells, and eliminates built-up waste and hardened material in the joints and muscles. It relieves pressure and irritation in the nerves, arteries and blood vessels and builds a healthy bloodstream. In summary it provides an overall boost to one's health.

Fasting is one of the oldest ways of healing and cleansing the body of diseases and build-up of mucus and toxins. Juice fasting helps restore the body to health as well as rejuvenates the system. It eliminates dead cells and toxic waste products that cause sickness and sluggish feelings. This method of fasting is safer than a water fast because poisons in the body are released into the blood stream more slowly. Some people fast anywhere from three to ten days.

Taking enemas is suggested during juice fasting by some nutritionist, for it helps assist the body in its cleansing and detoxifying effort by washing out all the toxic wastes from the alimentary canal. The following is a good example of what is commonly taken during a juice fast.

> 2 Tbsp. fresh lemon or lime juice
> 2 Tbsp. pure maple syrup
> 1/10 Tsp. cayenne pepper
> Pure Water: combine in 10 oz. hot or cold water
> Use 6 to 12 glasses daily

The lemon used in this diet is a loosening and cleansing agent with many important building factors. The ability of the elements in the lemon and the maple syrup, along with the cayenne pepper, work together for maximum benefit.

The natural iron, copper, calcium, carbon, and hydrogen found in the sweetening supplies more building and cleansing material. The cayenne pepper is necessary as it breaks up mucus and increases warmth by building the blood for an additional lift. It also adds many of the B vitamins and vitamin C. The following is a great example of a cleansing diet (there are various types). You can find many outstanding reference books that provide other effective cleansing diets.

If you become constipated, taking an herb laxative in the morning and evening is helpful. Also use lemon skin or pulp with the cleansing drink. Use mint tea to neutralize odors from the mouth.

Fasting is very beneficial, but it must be remembered that during a prolonged fast, the body is cleansing itself without any opportunity to replenish or regenerate the cells and tissues. (Read *Discover Your Fountain of Health* by Norman W. Walker, D. Sc.,

Ph.D.) The system is depleted of some of its most vital essential elements. Dr. Walker says that the immediate result of prolonged fasting is a feeling of well-being, but the damage to the system may not show up for one or two years longer. Therefore the safest way to fast would be to go on fruit juices for three to four days at a time, or no longer than six days, and then break the fast by drinking vegetable juices to build the body and also by eating raw vegetable and fruits for two or three days. This procedure can be repeated as long as it is felt necessary, but be sure and not fast more than six days. A mild food diet should follow a fast. This way you don't overload the system with hard-to-digest food.

A green drink is another excellent cleansing method and can be used to prepare for a fast. It is nourishing and very high in chlorophyll. I use this drink when I feel a cold coming on or when I feel that my body is full of toxins. In my favorite green drink, I use pineapple juice or fresh unfiltered apple juice, blended together with alfalfa sprouts, spearmint, parsley and comfrey.

## MILD FOOD DIET

A mild food diet is used in chronic sickness and for periodic cleansing. The following foods are recommended:

| | |
|---|---|
| Fruits, raw | Half fruit juice, half water |
| Vegetables, raw, | Vegetable juices |
| Raw cold pressed oils | Raw nuts |
| Honey, raw | Pure maple syrup |
| Seeds(sunflower, sesame) | Sprouts |
| Bake all starch vegetables | |

The following foods should be avoided during illness: grains, sugar, dairy products, butter, eggs, dried legume's, meats, peanuts, chips, soft drinks (including diet drinks).

## "GOOD-FOR-YOU" FOODS

*Fresh Raw Fruits:* Especially eaten in the season, where they are grown, full of vitamins and minerals

*Fresh Raw Vegetables:* Eat as many raw as possible or steam lightly.

*Fresh Raw Fruit Juices:* Wonderful used in a fast, full of enzymes, vitamins and minerals.

*Fresh Raw Vegetable Juices:* Living food, full of enzymes, vitamins and minerals.

*Yogurt, Kefir, Cottage Cheese Products:* Made with certified raw milk when possible.

*Kelp:* Contains iodine, use instead of salt.

*Cheeses:* Made naturally without artificial coloring and synthetic processing.

*Seeds:* Ground or sprouted, important to have sprouts on hand as they are living foods.

*Nuts:* Raw and fresh, keep in freezer to keep from getting rancid.

*Whole Grains:* Freshly ground when ready to use or sprouted for live enzymes.

*Honey:* Pure and natural, raw, full of vitamins and minerals, easily assimilated.

*Pure Maple Syrup:* Contains vitamins and minerals.

*Cold Pressed Oils:* Contains vitamin E, use with lemon juice or pure apple cider vinegar, use on salads.

*Fertile Eggs:* Contains protein and vitamins.

*Herbs:* Use garlic, capsicum, parsley, watercress, and paprika often.

*Dried Fruits:* Must be dried naturally in the sun with no chemicals added, should be soaked in water before eating to be more effective.

*Natural Sauerkraut:* Made at home fresh without chemicals with no salt added, very rich in calcium, and has great curative value.

*Herbal Teas:* Chamomile, licorice, spearmint and red raspberry

## NATURAL FOODS

The following are specific food items that are "natural," untainted by processing or manufacturing.

*Almonds:* high in protein, vitamin E, calcium

*Apples:* contains high levels of protein, enzymes and minerals. Useful for whatever ails you.

*Apricots:* is rich in minerals, especially iron. Detoxifies the liver and pancreas. High in vitamin A. Good for blood and skin, destroys worms.

*Avocados:* high in protein and fat. Good for the diabetic and hypoglycemic.

*Blackberries:* good for the colon and diarrhea.

*Blueberries:* nourishes the pancreas.

*Strawberries:* good for the skin, cleans the body and removes metallic poisons, such as arsenic.

*Carob Powder:* alkaline, contains minerals, a natural sweetner.

*Cherries:* cleanses intestines, minerals. Eat in season for one cleansing food diet. Also drink cherry juice.

*Citrus Fruits:* Vitamin C, use lemons, limes and pure water on occasional fasts. Cleanser, eliminates toxins. Juice of three lemons or limes in quart of warm water to drink during a fast. Helps eliminate the flu.

*Coconuts:* Supplies roughage.

*Dates:* high in protein, iron and mineral content, calcium and potassium.

*Figs:* contain iron, minerals, food for constipation.

*Fruits:* All fruits, very nourishing, especially when eaten in the season. Cleans and builds the body.

*Grains:* concentrated food, buckwheat, barley, millet, oats, rye and wheat. High in protein. Food for the vegetarian.

*Grapes:* Blood builder, good for anemia, antitumor food.

*Honey:* High in vitamins and minerals, use as substitute for white sugar. Use pure honey.

*Mustard Seeds:* Good for digestion and gas.

*Nut Butter:* More nourishing than dairy butter, grind fresh when ready to use.

*Nuts:* Raw, protein, unsaturated fats, minerals. Almonds, cashew, pecans, pistachio and walnuts.

*Oils:* Cold pressed are needed to assimilate the proteins from vegetables. Considered a kidney food.

*Papaya:* Good for digestion. Especially for protein foods.

*Seeds:* Contains the germ and embryo. Rich in oil, vitamin E. *Vitamin B-complex,* minerals and proteins.

*Sprouted Seeds:* Very healthy, the freshest food you can eat. Rich in enzymes, B-vitamins and hormones. Alfalfa, wheat, mung beans, radish, fenugreek, sunflower and chick peas are the most common and the best sprouted seeds.

*Sunflower Seeds:* Contain protein, vitamins and minerals. Feed the eyes, sinuses and glands.

*Vegetables:* High in enzymes, vitamins and minerals, carrot juice diluted is very good.

*Watercress:* Natural immune properties. High in vitamin A and C.

*Yogurt:* Beneficial for intestinal health.

# SECTION 6

# Special Uses
# of Herbs

# Herbs for Mothers
and Children

The best thing an expectant mother can do for her child is to obtain proper nutrition, exercise, fresh air, lots of pure water, sunshine, adequate sleep and relaxation. About 80 percent of the diet should be raw, natural food. Some of the best foods a pregnant woman can eat include grains (buckwheat, brown rice, whole wheat), nuts (almonds, pecans, piñons), seeds (sunflower, flax, pumpkin), and all types of vegetables and fruits.

## HERBS FOR MOTHERS

Herbs are also very helpful for dealing with some of the physical traumas of pregnancy. One herb that is especially known for its uses during pregnancy is red raspberry. It can be used as a tea or in capsule. It is safe and effective, strengthens the uterus for easier delivery and lessens bleeding during and after delivery. It is high in iron, and helps relieve "after-pain." Women who take red raspberry usually have shorter labors. The following subsections outline some of the ailments common to pregnancy and give their herbal and nutritional therapies.

## ANEMIA

Anemia is characterized by a lack of red blood cells, which are mainly responsible for transporting oxygen and nutrients to the body cells. Iron assists in this process, and is essential for improving one's anemic condition. Pregnant women need extra iron for this purpose. Yellow dock contains a high level of iron, as does red raspberry. This easy and tasty "green drink" recipe provides a large amount of natural iron. Combine either raw apple juice or pineapple juice with either comfrey, alfalfa sprouts, spearmint, or peppermint leaves, parsley and wheat grass. Blend in blender until smooth. Add about 500 mg of vitamin C, which helps iron absorb into the blood stream. Adding vitamin E can also help improve an anemic condition because it strengthens the blood cells.

## CONSTIPATION

For anyone who suffers from constipation, eating raw vegetables and fruits daily will inevitably help. Brewer's yeast and yogurt are useful for improving the growth of flora needed for proper digestion. Daily bran intake is especially effective for preventing constipation (remember to always drink large amounts of water when taking a bran supplement, as it can cause further constipation). Psyllium supplements or a lower bowel herbal formula can also be very helpful.

## FALSE LABOR

Drinking catnip as a tea in small amounts will help relieve false contractions. Blue cohosh is known to help relax the uterus, thereby preventing the false contractions.

## HEARTBURN

Papaya tablets can help relieve the sometimes severe heartburn that accompanies pregnancy. A combination of comfrey and pepsin can also help.

## INSOMNIA

Extra calcium can help improve sleep. The following herbal combination can also help decrease a tendency towards insomnia: comfrey, alfalfa, oat straw, Irish moss, horsetail, lobelia, and chamomile tea.

## MORNING SICKNESS

Teas made of red raspberry, catnip, peppermint or spearmint can help relieve nausea and morning sickness. Digestive enzymes can be helpful. Ginger is also widely known as an aid to nausea. Essential oils have also been useful.

## MISCARRIAGE

Taking red raspberry tea throughout the pregnancy can help prevent miscarriage. The following is a common uterine herbal combination used to prevent miscarriage: wild yam, squaw vine, false unicorn, and cramp bark. Lobelia and capsicum will help relax the uterus. Bayberry and catnip can help prevent miscarriage.

## TOXEMIA

A green drink is helpful in cleansing the circulatory system. Alfalfa, raspberry and comfrey tea is also cleansing and nourishing to the body. The following combinations are useful: (a) kelp, dandelion, and alfalfa; (b) red beet, yellow dock, strawberry, lobelia, burdock, nettle, and mullein. Stay away from red meat, white sugar products and white flour products. Add more vitamins A and C to your diet.

## OTHER

The following formulas will make the delivery and labor easier; it is suggested to start administering the formulas approximately six weeks before one's due date: (a) black cohosh, squaw vine, lobelia, pennyroyal, and red raspberry; (b) black cohosh, false unicorn, squaw vine, blessed thistle, lobelia, and red raspberry.

## NURSING MOTHERS

There are several herbs known to assist with the various ailments that a nursing mother can encounter. Refer to the following list.

*Nursing:* Blessed Thistle is know to increase mother's milk. Brewer's yeast taken daily will increase milk as well as give the mother necessary energy. Red raspberry and marshmallow tea is good. Alfalfa is excellent for rich milk and strength for the mother. Fennel seed boiled in barley water helps increase mother's milk.

*Breasts:* At first signs of breast becoming infected, take 1000 mgs of vitamin C every hour. Take extra vitamin A and E and garlic capsules. A green drink can also be very helpful for infections. For cracked, sore or dry nipples, apply thin honey or almond oil.

## HERBS FOR CHILDREN

*First Year of Life:* Fruit and vegetable juices of nut milks, always diluted. Raw apple juice and fresh carrot juice ar very nourishing. Vitamin C must be given, which is needed daily to build up resistance to germs. Babies need the amino acid (building blocks for body tissues) Taurine and mother's milk has a good supply but synthetic formulas don't. A deficiency of this amino acid in experiments has induced epileptic seizures. Taurine and B6 is a good combination for seizure problems.

*Colic:* Catnip tea has been used for years for colic in babies. Fennel and peppermint tea are good. Tincture of lobelia may be added to the tea.

*Constipation:* Small amount of mullein added to warm water, or weak licorice tea is good for babies. A nursing mother should watch her diet.

*Cradle Cap:* Vitamin E or almond oil rubbed into scalp.

*Digestion:* Difficulty in digesting cow's milk in children add powdered apple to milk or papaya.

*Diaper Rash:* Ground comfrey, goldenseal and make a paste with aloe vera juice. Vitamins E and A are good.

*Diarrhea:* Carob flour in pure water every few hours. Carob in boiled milk is good. Herb teas like those made of Red Raspberry, Slippery Elm, Ginger, Strawberry, Sage, Yarrow and Oak Bark are recommended.

*Dry Skin:* Olive oil, vitamin A and E and almond oil. Aloe vera is good.

*Ear Infection:* Garlic oil in ear. Garlic capsule in the rectum. Mullein oil, and lobelia extract.

*Fever:* Catnip tea, red raspberry or spearmint tea. Enemas help to bring fevers down.

*Hyperactivity:* Keep children away from sweets, artificial coloring, flavoring and preservatives. B-complex in water or juice, calcium herbal formula, vitamin D, multiple vitamin and mineral tablets are excellent for hyperactivity.

*Pinworms:* Raisins soaked in senna tea for older children is an old-time remedy. Chamomile and mint tea helps. Garlic in child's rectum will discard worms.

*Restlessness:* Chamomile tea, lobelia extract on the tongue will help relax the body.

*Teething:* Restless, crying babies who are teething need more calcium and vitamin D. Weak warm tea of catnip, chamomile, peppermint or fennel will help. Licorice root to chew on, it can dull the pain and irritation which teething causes.

*Sore Gums:* Rub the gums with thick honey to which a pinch of salt has been added. Honey with oil of chamomile, lobelia extract rubbed on gums and peppermint oil rubbed on gums will help.

*Urination Problems:* For infants who cannot urinate, administer crushed watermelon seeds in a tea. Give small amounts often.

# SECTION 7

# *Herbs and the Human Body*

# The Body Systems

Herbal medicines have been used with success for centuries. They are one of the oldest forms of therapy practiced by humans. Millions of people have testified to the benefits of herbal medicine. Approximately eighty percent of the world's population today depends on medicinal plants to heal and prevent disease.

The world's population, as well as its numerous physicians, are turning more and more to herbal medicines because they are considered safer than drugs. The side effects associated with the use of drugs are too numerous to mention. Drug companies are being sued constantly and settle out of court to prevent publicity.

Americans are becoming educated and more involved in their own health. We as individuals realize we have to take responsibility for our own health. Drugs will not heal the body—they just cause more problems and suppress the disease further in the system. Good health comes through learning more about diet, herbs, vitamins, minerals, and supplements that protect as well as help the body heal itself.

Currently, and in the past, doctors have said that herbs are unscientific, primitive, unproven, ineffective, possibly dangerous and do not have a place in our society today. This can no longer be said. There is now evidence of the validity of herbal medicine.

Science can now prove why herbs work to help the body heal itself. They are natural and do not cause side effects. When used with knowledge and guidance herbs strengthen, clean, nourish and stimulate body functions, and even prevent disease. We now know why the herbs work to heal the body. The following subsections give a brief overview of each of the body's systems along with the various disorders that commonly affect these systems, as well as herbal and nutritional supplements used to treat these disorders.

# THE CIRCULATORY SYSTEM

*H*eart disease is the number one killer of adults in the United States. Nearly one million people die each year of heart disease and related cardiovascular illness. Heart disease is striking people younger each year without warning and often fatal. It hits in many cases, without chest pains, shortness of breath or other symptoms common in heart disease. Cholesterol collects around the heart first then accumulates in the veins and arteries. This is why the heart can suffer damage first with out symptoms. These are related to bad diet, alcohol, smoking and lack of exercise. Lifestyle and diet change should be considered in order to protect the circulatory system. A typical American diet of meat and potatoes, sugar, and white flour products is paving the way for heart disease. A proper diet of whole grains (high fiber), fresh vegetables and fruits and herbs will clean and nourish the arteries.

Poor bowel function is another important cause of accumulation of fats and other toxins on the artery walls. It creates stagnation in the bowels, which fosters anaerobic bacteria that produce toxic waste. If the bowels are not properly eliminated after each meal. these toxins circulate in the blood stream and are deposited in the organs and other parts of the body.

# ORAL CHELATION FORMULA

An oral chelation formula that cleans the entire system and helps the blood flow more freely, improves circulation so that proper nutrition and oxidation can function in the body. The natural chelating elements work in a bonding reaction and surround the plaque, much like a magnet attracts metals. The chelation elements remove the built-up deposits on the arterial wall.

The natural chelation formula contains vitamins, minerals, glandular extracts, amino acids and herbs. It contains chelated minerals, a process where they are absorbed better by the body. It contains L-cysteine, HCL, choline, PABA, L-methionine, fish lipids, citrus bioflavonoids, rutin, adrenal substance, spleen extract, thymus substance, inositol. Hawthorn berries and ginkgo biloba are two herbs beneficial for circulation. It contains vitamins A, D, E, C, B1, B2, B6, B12, niacin, pantothenic acid, folic acid, biotin magnesium, iron, iodine, copper and zinc. It also contains chromium, selenium, potassium, manganese and calcium.

# BLOOD PURIFYING FORMULAS

Impurities in the blood affect the heart. The toxins are collected by both the blood and the lymph fluid that pass through the heart continually. It is important to purify the blood. The following formulas will help purify the blood stream.

#1. Red Clover, Chaparral, Spice

#2. Ganoderma, Dang Gui, Peony, Lycium, Bupleurum, Curcuma, Cornus, Saliva, Ho Shu Wu, Atractylodes, Achranthes, Ligustrum, Alisma, Astragalus, Ligusticum, Rehmannia, Panax Ginseng, Cyperus

#3. Pau D'Arco, Red Clover, Yellow Dock, Burdock, Sarsaparilla, Dandelion, Chaparral, Cascara Sagrada, Buckthorn, Peach Bark, Barberry, Stillingia, Prickly Ash, Yarrow

## CIRCULATORY SYSTEM ENHANCERS

#1. This formula will provide nutrients to the eyes, ears, and nose areas to clean and nourish: Goldenseal, Bayberry, Eyebright, Red Raspberry.

#2. This formula increases resistance to stress with it natural nutrients to enhance the circulatory, glandular, and nervous systems: Siberian Ginseng, Bee pollen, Yellow Dock, Licorice, Gotu, Kola, Kelp, Schizandra, Barley Grass, Rose hips, Capsicum.

#3. This formula feeds and strengthens the heart: Hawthorn Berries, Capsicum, Garlic.

#4. This Chinese formula is known to nourish the heart, and strengthen the circulatory system: Schizandra, Dang Gui (Dong Quai), Cistanche, Biota, Succinum, Ophiopogon, Cuscuta, Lycium, Panax, Ginseng, Polygonum, Hoelen, Dioscorea, Astragalus, Lotus, Polygala, Acorus, Zizyphus, Rehmannia.

#5. This stimulates circulation and elimination which has a positive affect on the immune system: Garlic, Capsicum, Parsley, Siberian Ginseng, Goldenseal.

#6. This formula contains Ginkgo and Hawthorn. The Ginkgo protects the cells of the body and especially those of the brain. It increases circulation, to deliver oxygen and glucose to the cells. It protects against free radical damage, and protects the nervous system.

#7. Capsicum, Garlic and Parsley are also beneficial to nourish the heart. Parsley is a natural diuretic, and rich in minerals. Garlic helps to dissolve cholesterol plaque on the artery walls. It stimulates lymphatic system to eliminate toxins and is a natural antibiotic.

#8. This formula is rich in iron for healthy blood: Red Beet Root, Yellow Dock, Red Raspberry, Chickweed, Burdock, Nettle, Mullein.

## OTHER HERBS AND SUPPLEMENTS

The following are single herbal and supplemental products that have shown beneficial qualities for improving cardiovascular health.

*Omega-3 Fatty Acid:* An essential nutrient for the body. It helps the body create a hormone-type substance called prostacyclin. This prevents blood cells from sticking together and decreases the danger of blood clots producing strokes and heart attacks.

*Coenzyme Q-10 Formula:* Contains the minerals copper, iron, magnesium and zinc and the amino acids leucine, histidine and glycine and the herbs capsicum and hawthorn. This formula increases oxygen to the brain and cells, prevents circulatory problems. Strengthens the heart and immune system.

*Liquid Chlorophyll:* Repairs tissues. Helps to neutralize pollution that we eat and breathe. It helps in the assimilation of calcium and other minerals. Purifies and strengthens the entire body.

*Suma, Astragalus, Siberian Ginseng, Ginkgo and Gotu Kola:* A powerhouse of herbs to increase circulation, feed and strengthen the brain, eyes, ears, nose and throat. Improves memory, alertness, and an overall good feeling of well-being.

*L-Carnitine:* Energizes the body, effective in lowering cholesterol, cleans the veins and arteries and strengthens the muscles, especially the heart. It burns fat, and reduces built-up fat in the body. Cleans the veins and strengthens the muscles, especially the heart.

*Other single herbs for the circulatory system:* Aloe Vera, Bilberry, Bugleweed, Butcher's Broom, Cayenne, Cloves, Garlic, Ginger, Ginkgo, Hawthorn, Horseradish, Prickly Ash, Suma, Virginia Snake Root

# THE DIGESTIVE SYSTEM

*D*igestive disorders are one of the most common health problems that plague people today. Both the old and the young are having more digestive problems. Improper digestion can cause poor assimilation, especially essential minerals. Lack of minerals and essential fatty acids can produce unhealthy cells. Digestive upsets are mainly caused by stress, constipation, faulty diet, drugs, alcohol and tobacco. Eating wholesome, natural food nourishes the digestive system and strengthens the whole body.

## DIGESTIVE FORMULA

This formula is more than a digestive aid; it works with the liver, gallbladder, and spleen to promote normal function of the digestive system. This will also benefit the lymphatic and urinary systems. It helps in the production of bile which digests fat and prevents constipation. It helps with gas and bloating, fluid retention, digestion and in the assimilation of nutrients.

#1. Rose Hips, Barberry, Dandelion, Fennel, Red Beet Root, Horseradish, Parsley

#2. Protein Digestive Aid: Production of hydrochloric acid (HCL) decreases as people age. It is essential for the breakdown of proteins, starches and many foods. Hydroclyric acid destroys harmful bacteria. Worms and parasites are destroyed by HCL.

#3. Digestive enzymes are necessary for digestion of proteins, fats and carbohydrates. Enzymes are essential for proper digestion. All food needs enzymes to be broken down into simple building blocks. Enzymes are destroyed by heating, emotional stress, drugs and toxins we eat and breathe.

## DIGESTIVE SYSTEM FORMULAS

These formulas improve digestion and most ailments are benefited when digestion is strengthened. These herbs help to calm a nervous stomach, aid digestion, provide enzymes and protein digestive aids.

#1. This is a Chinese formula which enhances the digestive system and also benefits the urinary system in the elimination of toxins. It will help prevent nausea, gas, bloating, allergies, motion sickness and craving for sweets. It includes: Magnolia, Shenqu Tea, Crataegus, Oryza, Hoelen, Panax Ginseng, Pinellia, Saussurea, Gastrodia, Citrus, Atractylodes, Cardamon, Platycodon, Ginger, Licorice.

#2. Papaya, Ginger, Peppermint, Wild Yam, Fennel, Dong Quai, Spearmint, Catnip

#3. Barberry, Ginger, Cramp Bark, Fennel, Peppermint, Wild Yam, Catnip

#4. Red Beet Root, Dandelion, Parsley, Horsetail, Liverwort, Black Cohosh, Birch, Blessed Thistle, Angelica, Chamomile, Gentian, Goldenrod

#5. Papaya and Mint

#6. Goldenseal, Juniper, Uva Ursi, Cedar Berries, Mullein, Yarrow, Garlic, Slippery Elm, Capsicum, Dandelion, Marshmallow, Nettle, White Oak Bark, Licorice

#7. This formula benefits the stomach and the intestinal system. It helps prevent indigestion, infections, inflammations, ulcers, and toxic accumulation: Slippery Elm, Marshmallow, Dong Quai, Ginger, and Wild Yam.

#8. This Chinese formula is very beneficial to the digestive and nervous systems. This will benefit in many health problems. When the nerves are strengthened it fortifies the immune system. This also benefits the urinary and intestinal systems. It includes: Bupleurum, Peony, Pinellia, Cinnamon, Dang Gui (Dong Quai) Fushen, Zhishi, Scute, Atractylodes, Panax Ginseng, Ginger, and Licorice.

#9. This is another beneficial Chinese formula that works with the digestive system. This strengthens digestion to prevent indigestion, colitis, poor circulation and many health problems that go along with an unbalanced center of digestion. It includes: Panax Ginseng, Astragalus, Atractylodes, Hoelen, Dioscorea, Lotus, Galanga, Pinellia, Chaenomeles, Magnolia, Saussurea, Dang Gui (Dong Quai), Citrus Peel, Dolichos, Licorice, Ginger, Zanthoxylum, and Cardamon.

#10. This combination will strengthen and heal the digestive and intestinal systems. It includes: Ginger, Capsicum, Goldenseal, Licorice.

## SINGLE HERBS FOR THE DIGESTIVE SYSTEM

Alfalfa, provides essential minerals and aids digestion. Aloe Vera heals and protects the mucous membranes, will heal ulcers and even scars from adhesion. Buchu heals the digestive tract, absorbs excessive uric acid and acts as a tonic. Capsicum, heals and stops internal bleeding, acts as a disinfectant and aids in digestion. Other beneficial herbs include comfrey, fennel, gentian, ginger, papaya, parsley, peppermint, and slippery elm.

# THE GLANDULAR SYSTEM

The glandular or endocrine system consists of the pituitary gland, thyroid gland, parathyroid gland, thymus gland, sex glands (ovaries, testes), pancreas, hypothalamus and adrenal glands. Along with the nervous system, hormones, the secretions of the glands of the glandular system, are the major means of controlling the body's activities. The glandular system has a direct effect upon mood, mind, behavior, immune defense, memory, control of metabolic rate, and control of blood sugar to name a few.

All the glands depend upon one another and work together synergistically. The glandular system is necessary for survival, a healthy system is essential for health. An imbalance in any gland of the glandular system will cause enormous problems for the entire body. There are many problems that can happen because of glandular imbalance. Vitamins, minerals and herbs nourish and restore glandular health.

## GLANDULAR FORMULA

This was formulated to nourish and strengthen the entire glandular system. The nutrients of vitamins, minerals and herbs are combined with necessary essential ingredients to stimulate proper hormone production and metabolism.

Vitamin A nourishes the thymus gland, as well as all the glands, to increase its size and antibody production. Zinc protect the immune system and supports the T-cells. Low zinc intake decreases thymus growth. Lecithin breaks down fatty deposits, especially effective on the liver. Vitamin C nourishes and cleans all the glands and with the lemon bioflavonoids, helps protect the immune system. The minerals, especially the trace minerals in the herbs, are vital for glandular health. Kelp is rich in iodine and contains all essential minerals. Alfalfa is rich in minerals and eliminates uric acid from the body. Parsley is a natural diuretic and eliminates toxins such as uric acid. Dandelion stimulates bile production and benefits the spleen and pancreas. Licorice root strengthens the adrenal, pancreas and spleen.

## HERBAL FORMULAS FOR THE GLANDULAR SYSTEM

#1. This formula enhances the glandular system. It is especially beneficial for the pancreas in the production of pancretin and bile from the gallbladder. It also helps improve liver function, and is also beneficial for the urinary system. This formula includes: Cedar Berries, Burdock, Chaparral, Goldenseal, and Siberian Ginseng.

#2. This formula strengthens the digestive system. Lack of proper digestion can cause malfunction of the glands. The formula includes: Barberry, Ginger, Cramp Bark, Fennel, Peppermint, Wild Yam, and Catnip.

#3. This formula nourishes the pancreas, liver, adrenals and the digestive system. It includes: Licorice, Safflower, Dandelion, and Horseradish.

#4. This formula provides nutrition especially for the thyroid, but is beneficial for all the gland because of the complete mineral content. The minerals help eliminate toxic metal and poisons from the body. The formula includes: Irish Moss, Kelp, Black Walnut, Parsley, Watercress, and Sarsaparilla.

#5. This formula helps bile production to digest fat and prevent constipation. It nourishes the liver, gallbladder, digestive system, spleen, immune system as well as the glandular system: Rose Hips, Barberry, Dandelion, Fennel, Red Beet Root, Horseradish, and Parsley.

#6. This formula is designed to feed the liver. The liver is vital to detoxify the system. A healthy liver is important to the glandular system. The formula includes: Red Beet Root, Dandelion, Parsley, Horsetail, and Liverwort.

#7. This formula nourishes the glandular system, especially the pancreas and prostate. It includes: Goldenseal, Juniper, Uva Ursi, Cedar Berries, Mullein, Yarrow, Garlic, Slippery Elm, Capsicum, Dandelion, Marshmallow, Nettle, White Oak Bark, and Licorice.

#8. This formula is rich in minerals to five nutritional support to the glandular system, especially the hypothalamus and thyroid glands. These contain chelated minerals for easy absorption to benefit specific body systems. It includes: Zinc, Manganese, Kelp, Irish Moss, Parsley, Hops, and Capsicum.

#9. This formula helps balance the glandular system. It is rich in iodine, iron, calcium and magnesium. It includes: Kelp, Dandelion, and Alfalfa.

#10. This is a formula to benefit the glandular system especially the thyroid, the master gland. The hops are added to control the stress of the system. Stress depletes nutrients, and this will add extra nutrients to protect the glands. It includes: Kelp, Irish Moss, Parsley, Hops, and Capsicum.

#11. This formula is designed to nourish the glandular, nervous and circulatory systems. This is a natural way to provide the body with nutrients that help it adapt to stress. The formula includes: Siberian Ginseng, Bee Pollen, Yellow Dock, Licorice, Gotu Kola, Kelp, Schizandra, Barley Grass, Rose Hips, and Capsicum.

#12. This formula is to support the glandular system when the body is undergoing fasting or cleansing programs. It will help nourish, strengthen and fortify the glands when under stress. It includes: Chickweed, Cascara Sagrada, Licorice, Safflower, Parthenium, Black walnut, Gotu Kola, Hawthorn, Papaya, Fennel, and Dandelion.

#13. This formula is excellent for athletes. It provides the body with nutrients not only for athletes but for andy one who is active in physical stress. It could also help parents who are active with children. It includes: Siberian Ginseng, Ho Shou Wu, Black Walnut, Licorice, Gentian, Fennel, Slippery Elm, Bee Pollen, Bayberry, Myrrh, Peppermint, Safflower, Eucalyptus, Lemon Grass, and Capsicum.

#14. This formula is to help the body maintain a balance in weight control. Along with a high fiber diet, using whole grains, fruits and vegetables and natural supplements, this formula will help in weight control. It includes: Licorice, Red Beet Root, Hawthorn, and Fennel.

#15. This formula is for an over-stressed body, where the glands become weakened and puts stress on the entire body. This will give the body nutrients essential for the energy it needs to function properly. The formula includes: Suma, Astragalus, Siberian Ginseng, Ginkgo, and Gotu Kola.

#16. This formula is designed to support the nutritional needs of the pancreas: Chromium, Zinc, Goldenseal, Juniper, Uva Ursi, Huckleberry, Mullein, Yarrow, Garlic, Slippery Elm, Capsicum, Dandelion, Marshmallow, Nettle, White Oak, and Licorice.

#17. This is a Chinese formula that is very beneficial to strengthen the glandular system. When the glands are out of balance it can cause a number of health problems. It includes: Dendrobium, Eucommia, Rehmannia, Ophiopogon, Trichosanthes, Pueraria, Anemarrhena, Achyranthes, Hoelen, Asparagus, Moutan, Alisma, Phellondendron, Cornus, Licorice, and Schizandra.

## FEMALE GLANDS

This female glandular formula contains vitamins, minerals and herbs to provide nutritional support and prevent deficiencies that cause emotional and physical symptoms and problems common to women. This nutritional support will help prevent physical and mental stress which causes fatigue, depression, irritability, and chemical imbalances which can lead to a dependency on antidepressant drugs.

It contains vitamins A, C, B1, B2, niacinamide, vitamin D, E, B6, folic acid, B12, biotin, pantothenic acid; minerals, calcium, iron, iodine, magnesium, zinc, copper, manganese, chromium, selenium and potassium. It also contains choline, inositol, bioflavonoids, and PABA. It also contains the following Chinese herbs: dong quai, peony, bupleurum, hoelen, atractylodes, codonopsis, alisma, licorice, magnolia, ginger, peppermint, moutan, gardenia and cyperus.

## FEMALE FORMULAS

#1. This is designed to help maintain the female glands as well as other glands. This will nourish and strengthen the reproductive glands and prevent menstrual pain, premenstrual tension, insomnia, menopausal symptoms, sexual disinterest and other problems that are caused by chemical imbalance. It includes: Black Cohosh, Licorice, Siberian Ginseng, Sarsaparilla, Squaw vine, Blessed Thistle, and False Unicorn.

#2. This formula is designed to help prepare a woman for giving birth by strengthening the glands and reproductive systems. This supplies nutrients to build a weakened body, to prevent menstrual disorders, morning sickness, miscarriage, as well as menopausal symptoms. It includes: Black Cohosh, Squaw Vine, Dong Quai, Butcher's Broom, and Red Raspberry.

#3. This is formulated especially for the female reproductive organs and also benefits the glandular system. This is rich in herbs that contain vitamins and minerals that feed and strengthen the female glands. The formula includes: Red Raspberry, Dong Quai, Ginger, Licorice, Black Cohosh, Queen of the Meadow, Blessed Thistle, and Marshmallow.

#4. This is designed to strengthen the female reproductive system and the urinary system. This helps to prevent cramps, bloating, morning sickness, and menstrual disorders. It includes: Goldenseal, Red Raspberry, Black Cohosh, Queen of the Meadow, Althea, Blessed Thistle, Dong Quai, Capsicum, and Ginger.

#5. This is a nutritional herbal supplement to help balance hormones, prevent bad estrogen from accumulating, bloating, post partum problems, weakness in the veins, hemorrhaging, anemia, and strengthen the urinary system. It includes: Goldenseal,

Capsicum, Ginger, Uva Ursi, Cramp Bark, Squaw vine, Blessed Thistle, Red Raspberry, and False Unicorn.

#6. A liquid formula for easy digestion and assimilation. It enhances nutritional support for the digestive and glandular systems. It includes: Peppermint, Rose Hips, Hibiscus, and Red Raspberry.

## MALE FORMULAS

#1. A special formula for the prostate gland as well as for the glandular system. This will help balance hormones in the body. It helps to supply nutrients for inflammation and pain in the prostate gland. It includes: Black Cohosh, Licorice, Kelp, Gotu Kola, Capsicum, Goldenseal, Ginger, and Dong Quai.

#2. A special formula for the male reproductive system as well as beneficial for the urinary system. Nutrients to help prevent kidney stones, inflammation, infections, impotence, edema, joint pain, prostatitis. The formula includes: Capsicum, Goldenseal, Ginger, Parsley, Siberian Ginseng, Uva Ursi, Marshmallow, and Eupatorium.

#3. This is especially formulated for the male reproductive system. It provides nutrients to nourish and strengthen the prostate. It helps prevent swelling, inflammation and prevent pain. This is important for older men, who need nutrients for proper function of the male glands. It includes: Siberian Ginseng, Parthenium, Saw Palmetto, Gotu Kola, Damiana, Sarsaparilla, Horsetail, Garlic, Capsicum, and Chickweed.

#4. This formula is designed to help strengthen the glandular system, especially for the pancreas and prostate. It helps in infections, water retention and supplies circulation to prevent toxins form accumulating in the glands. The formula includes:

Single Herbs for the Male Glands, Black Walnut, Damiana, Ho Shou Wu, Sarsaparilla, Saw Palmetto, Siberian Ginseng, American Ginseng, and Suma.

# THE IMMUNE SYSTEM

The immune system is a network of mechanisms and processes that keep us safe from bacteria, viruses, yeast/fungi infections and any other toxins that may invade our tissues. The immune system accumulates damage, and gradually becomes defective over many years and is implicated in the autoimmune diseases that are prevalant now. Diet and lifestyle have a profound effect on the immune system. Evidence has been produced that shows how stress, and how we cope with stress, are the main causes of illness.

Stress effects the body by depleting the adrenal glands. This causes a suppressed immune system. This happens because the immune system requires enormous amounts of nutrients. The body also requires large amounts of nutrients and the average American diet does not supply the body's needs. Our food is processed, with added chemicals, food coloring, preservatives and taste enhancers. The natural food is processed and depleted of the vital vitamins such a B-vitamins and minerals that are essential for a healthy immune system.

Viruses are composed of living and nonliving material. They can be dormant for years and if the immune system is weak, come to life. The virus inserts its genetic material through the cell wall. It then dissolves the wall and fuses with the contents of the cell, and thus multiplies and begins to do its damage.

## IMMUNE FORMULA

This formula contains nutrients to protect and strengthen the immune system. It contains the necessary ingredients for a healthy immune system to fight toxins, germs and viruses that constantly invade our bodies. The formula includes the following: Vitamin A from fish oils and beta carotene, Vitamin C, Vitamin E, Zinc and Selenium. Barley Grass Juice Powder, Wheat Grass Juice Powder, Asparagus Powder, Astragalus, Broccoli Powder, Cabbage Powder, Ganoderma, Parthenium, Schizandra, Siberian Ginseng, Myrrh Gum, and Pau d'Arco.

## SPECIAL IMMUNE FORMULAS

#1. This formula was designed to nourish and strengthen the immune system. It also protects the body against stress and gives the body a feeling of well-being. This will aid in healing as well as protect against viruses that cause autoimmune diseases. The formula includes: Rose Hips, Beta Carotene, Broccoli Powder, Cabbage Powder, Siberian Ginseng, Parsley Red Clover, Wheat Grass Powder, and Horseradish.

#2. This formula is beneficial for the immune an circulatory systems. This help protect against germs and viruses that cause illness. It includes: Rose Hips, Chamomile, Slippery Elm, Yarrow, Capsicum, Goldenseal, Myrrh Gum, Peppermint, Sage, and Lemon Grass.

#3. This not only strengthens the immune system but aids in digestion and the lymph system. It helps in fever, vomiting, motion sickness, chills, abdominal pain, and water retention. It includes: Ginger, Capsicum, Goldenseal, and Licorice.

#4. Germanium is an antioxidant which neutralizes free radicals to prevent them from damaging tissues in the body. Echinacea helps neutralizes toxins and rid them from the body. It includes: Germanium and Echinacea.

#5. This formula aids the body from stress that weakens the immune system. It also is beneficial for the lymphatic and respiratory systems. It includes: Parthenium, Yarrow, Myrrh Gum, and Capsicum.

#6. This formula is an immune system enhancer. It helps purify the lymphatic and strengthen the digestive system. It helps in infections, colds flu and with swollen glands. The formula includes: Parthenium, Yarrow, Myrrh Gum, and Capsicum.

#7. This formula strengthens the eliminative system which can cause a weakened immune system. A weak immune system will open the door to all kinds of illness. This formula includes: Goldenseal, Black Walnut, Althea (Marshmallow), Parthenium, Plantain, and Bugleweed.

#8. Red Clover Formula. This formula helps purify and eliminate toxins, germs and viruses from the body. It is also useful in liquid form for easy assimilation for those who have faulty digestion. The formula includes: Red Clover, Chaparral, Spice.

#9. This formula is designed to strengthen the immune system. This contains chelated minerals which are necessary to enzymes for the immune system such as superoxide dismutase (SOD). The formula includes: Vitamin A (beta carotene), Copper, Manganese, Zinc.

#10. This formula is designed to fortify and strengthen the body to protect against yeast infestations and other microorganisms that invade when the immune system is weak. This provides nutrients to strengthen and protect the immune system. The formula includes: Caprylic Acid, Vitamin A, E, C, Pantothenic Acid, Biotin, Zinc, Selenium.

#11. This formula is designed to protect and build up the immune system. It contains nutrients that are vital for the protection of the immune system. The minerals have been chelated to specific amino acids glutamine and glycine. This provides for better assimilation. The formula includes: Vitamin A (beta carotene), Copper, Manganese, Zinc, Barley Green Juice Powder.

#12. A combination of Goldenseal and Parthenium in an extract form is designed to heal and strengthen the immune system and protect against diseases. Goldenseal is the greatest healer in the herbal kingdom. It will heal and repair the entire digestive tract. Parthenium will help the lymphatic system to keep the body clean.

#13. This Chinese formula is carefully designed to strengthen the immune system. It protects against viral infections, and protects against germs. The formula includes: Dandelion, Purslane, Indigo, Thlaspi, Bupleurum, Scute, Pinella, Ginseng, Cinnamon, Licorice.

#14. This Chinese formula is designed to increase circulation, which helps fight and prevent infections. It will strengthen the immune system by stimulating circulation, which is the key to a healthy body. The formula includes: Astragalus, Panax Ginseng, Dang Qui (Dong Quai), Rehmannia, Epimedim, Ganoderm, Eucommia, Lycium, Peony, Polygala, Ligustrum, Schizandra, Atractylodes, Hoelen, Achyranthes, Ophiopogon, Citrus Peel, Licorice.

#15. This formula is in an extract for quicker assimilation to quicker action. It strengthens the immune and nervous systems. This is useful to help fight infections, especially for all kinds of ear problems, such as ear infections, accumulation of wax in the ears, itching ears, and has been used for some types of hearing loss. It can also be used for throat infections. The formula includes: Black

Cohosh, Chickweed, Goldenseal, Desert Tea, Licorice, Valerian, Skullcap.

### SINGLE HERBS FOR THE IMMUNE SYSTEM

Single herbs that are known to assist in building and maintaining a healthy immune system include the following: Barley Juice Powder, Blue Vervain, Burdock, Chaparral, Echinacea, Ginkgo, Goldenseal, Parthenium, Pau d'Arco, Rose Hips, and Suma.

# THE INTESTINAL SYSTEM

The colon is the body's sewer system, and if not treated properly can accumulate toxic poisons, which are absorbed into the blood stream. This will then cause many diseases. Lack of fiber in the diet is the main cause of intestinal diseases. Years of poor diet cause bowel problems.

The small intestine is where most nutrition is absorbed. Stress can affect nutrients absorption and cause irritation of the small intestine. The large intestine absorbs minerals and water. When the membrane of the large colon is unhealthy, it cannot assimilate and absorb the minerals and creates deficiency diseases. The health of the entire body is maintained when the intestinal system is working properly.

## HERBAL FORMULAS

### BOWEL FORMULA

This formula benefits the entire gastrointestinal tract. It supplies nutrients for a healthy colon. It strengthens and heals the stomach, nourishes and cleans the intestines, stimulates bile function and liver health. It dissolves and eliminates mucus from the intestinal tract. It contains nutrients for proper digestion and assimilation.

It contains betaine HCL, pepsin, pancreatin and bile salts for upper gastrointestinal system. It contains psyllium hulls, kelp and chlorophyll to clean and nourish the lower bowels. It also contains vitamin C, E and beta carotene, selenium and zinc. It contains algin, cascara sagrada, bentonite clay, apple pectin, marshmallow root, parthenium root, charcoal, ginger, and sodium copper chlorophyllin.

## GYMNEMA FORMULA

Excellent for the digestive and glandular systems. Research on gymnema shows good results on nourishing the pancreas and helping with problems such as diabetes, obesity and glandular problems. The formula includes: Brindall Berries, Gymnema Leaves, Marshmallow, Psyllium Hulls.

## PUMPKIN SEED FORMULA

This formula is good for parasites, cleans the colon, skin problems, removes toxins from the system, constipation, prostate, tumors, worms. The formula includes: Pumpkin Seeds, Culvers Root, Cascara Sagrada, Violet, Chamomile, Mullein, Marshmallows, and Slippery Elm.

## LOWER BOWEL FORMULAS

The herbs in these formulas tone, rebuild and strengthen the bowels. They will gradually clean and restore bowel function. Constipation causes poisons to accumulate in the blood and prevents food from being assimilated.

#1. This formula is designed to help the entire intestinal tract. This will enhance normal liver function. It strengthens the gall bladder, urinary and lymphatic systems. The formula includes: Rose Hips, Barberry, Dandelion, Fennel, Red Beet Root, Horseradish, Parsley.

#2. This formula will help heal and restore normal lower bowel function. It will also also help purify the blood. The formula includes: Cascara Sagrada, Buckthorn, Licorice, Capsicum, Ginger, Barberry, Turkey Rhubarb, Couch Grass, Red Clover.

#3. This formula is rich in fiber and minerals for the lower bowels. It helps restore normal function to weakened bowels. The formula includes: Dong Quai, Cascara Sagrada, Turkey Rhubarb, Goldenseal, Capsicum, Ginger, Barberry, Fennel, Red Raspberry.

#4. This formula contains nature's natural fibers. It will absorb toxins and rid them from the body. It will help lower cholesterol. It is a natural way to retore normal bowel function. The formula includes: Psyllium, Oat, Apple Fibers.

#5. This formula is an excellent way to clean the bowels. The ginger helps prevent any cramps due to the Senna. The catnip helps relax the bowels, and the formula is rich in minerals, which are absorbed in the lower bowels. The formula includes: Senna Leaves, Fennel, Ginger, Catnip.

#6. This formula works on the lower bowels to promote the friendly bacteria, essential for a healthy colon. This is soothing and healing to the entire intestinal system. The formula includes: Slippery Elm, Marshmallow, Plantain, Chamomile, Rose hips, Bugleweed.

#7. This Chinese formula helps detoxify and clean the intestinal system. The formula includes: Ionicera, Scute, Forsythia, Platycodon, Ligusticum, Schizonepeta, Peony, Chrysanthemum, Gardenia, Phellodendron, Siler, Bupleurum, Dang Qui (Dong Quai), Arctium, Vitex, Licorice, Carthamus, Coptis.

## GENERAL CLEANSING FORMULA

This formula benefits the colon, blood and cells of the body. It is an excellent formula to use on a weight loss program. It is an excellent blood cleanser to use for any disease.

#1. Gentian, Irish Moss, Cascara Sagrada, Goldenseal, Slippery Elm, Fenugreek, Safflower, Myrrh, Yellow Dock, Parthenium, Black Walnut, Barberry, Dandelion, Uva Ursi, Chickweed, Catnip, Cyani

### SUPPLEMENTS AND SINGLE HERBS

Acidophilus, Aloe Vera, Hydrated, Bentonite, Liquid Chlorophyll, Magnesium, Black walnut, Buckthorn, Cascara Sagrada, Chaparral, Dandelion, Fennel, Fenugreek, Flax, Ginger, Goldenseal, Licorice, marshmallow, Oregon Grape, Peppermint, Psyllium, Safflowers, Sarsaparilla, Senna Vervain, Slippery Elm

# THE NERVOUS SYSTEM

The nervous system is a very delicate and important part of the body and needs to be treated properly. The nervous system and the immune system are closely connected. When one system fails the other is affected. The brain has the job of transmitting information back and forth from the immune system. It is vital to nourish and strengthen the nervous system in order to protect the immune system.

## STRESS FORMULA

Stressful situations leach out nutrients from the body. Nutritionist regard inadequate nutrients as the most stressful on the immune system as well as the nervous system. This formula is designed to fortify the body against depleted essential nutrients and protect the body under stress. It contains Vitamin C, B1, B2, B6, B12, Folic Acid, Biotin, Niacinamide, Pantothenic Acid, schizandra, Choline Bitartrate, PABA, Wheat Germ, Bee Pollen, Valerian Root, Skullcap, Inositol, Hops, Citrus Bioflavonoids.

## HERBAL FORMULAS FOR THE NERVES

#1. This formula is designed to relax the nerves and nourish and strengthen the nervous system. It is especially good for spastic colon and muscle spasms. It helps prevent migraine headaches. It is rich in calcium and B-complex vitamins which provides nutritional support for the nervous system. The formula includes: Chamomile, Passionflower, Hops, Fennel, Marshmallow, Feverfew.

#2. This formula is designed to strengthen weakened nerves and help in nervous tension, Cramps, Headaches, Hysteria, pain and insomnia. This will build the nerves to help in coughs, cramps, vertigo, and with colds, flu and fevers. The formula includes: White Willow, Valerian, Lettuce leaves, and Capsicum.

#3. A formula to strengthen the nervous system as well as cleansing power to clean the muscles and tissues. The Devil's claw works similar to Chaparral and enhances this formula. The formula includes: White Willow, Black Cohosh, Capsicum, Valerian, Ginger, Hops, Wood Betony, Devil's Claw.

#4. This is formulated for an over-stressed nervous system. It helps with insomnia, hypertension, menstrual disorders, nervous indigestion, headache, epilepsy, arthritis and rheumatism. The formula includes: Valerian, Skullcap, Hops.

#5. This formula not only strengthens the nervous system but benefits peripheral blood circulation. It helps relieve anxiety and tense muscles. It will gradually build a strong nervous system which protects the immune system. Valerian is rich in calcium and the passion flower is beneficial for the eyes. The formula includes: Black Cohosh, Valerian, Capsicum, Passionflower, Skullcap, Hops, Wood Betony.

#6. This Chinese formula is beneficial on the nervous system. It helps to prevent depression, insomnia, fatigue, anxiety, and menopause symptoms. It also strengthens the urinary, respiratory and female reproductive systems. The formula includes: Perilla, Saussurea, Gambir, Bamboo Sap, Bupleurum, Pinellia, Aurantium, Zhishi, Ophiopogon, Cyperus, Platycodon, Liqusticum, Dand Gui, Panax, Ginseng, Hoelen, Coptis, Ginger, Licorice.

#7. An extract formula which is used to calm, nourish, and strengthen the nervous system. It is useful for those who need to build up their digestive system. It is easily assimilated and contains minerals to build up the digestive and nervous system. It can be used under the tongue with quick results. The formula includes: Valerian, Anise, Black Walnut, Desert Tea, Ginger, Licorice.

#8. This Chinese formula contains nutrients vital for a strong nervous system. It also benefits the digestive and urinary systems. The formula includes: Dragon Bone, Oyster Shell, Albizzia, Polygonum, Fushen, Polygala, Acorus, Panax Ginseng, Saussurea, Zizphus, Curcuma, Haliotis Shell, Coptis, Cinnamon, Licorice, Ginger.

#9. This combination supplies nutrients that strengthen the nervous system. It also benefits the respiratory and muscle systems. The formula includes: Blessed Thistle, Pleurisy, Skullcap, Yerba Santa.

## SINGLE HERBS FOR THE NERVES

Bilberry, Black Currant Oil, Catnip, Chaparral, Feverfew, Hops, Lady's Slipper, Passionflower, Skullcap, Valerian, Wood Betony

# THE RESPIRATORY SYSTEM

Respiratory infections are the most frequent single cause of illness. One-third to one-half of industrial absenteeism from sickness is caused by acute respiratory illness. The lungs have the responsibility of supplying oxygen necessary for body energy. Toxins present in the atmosphere, such as nitrogen and ozone dioxide, are increasing as a major cause of respiratory problems. Pollutants can attack the body repeatedly over a long period before symptoms appear. The respiratory system consists of the lungs, nose, throat and trachea.

Herbs, vitamins, minerals and proper diet will help keep the respiratory system strong and healthy. A colon cleanse is essential for a healthy respiratory system.

## RESPIRATORY FORMULA

This formula was developed for severe lung congestion, allergies, lungs filling with fluid, mucus, pneumonia, coughs and toxic build-up in the lungs. It also helps in digestion. The herbs in this formula will help protect the lungs from all the pollutants in the air. It helps loosen hard mucus from the sinuses, throat, and lungs. It will help in asthma, bronchitis, coughs, hayfever, nasal drainage, earache, sinus swelling and swollen glands. The formula includes: Boneset, Fenugreek, Horseradish, Mullein, Fennel.

## SPECIAL RESPIRATORY FORMULAS

#1. This Chinese formula is beneficial for the respiratory system. It also helps with the circulatory and lymphatic systems. It increases circulation and eliminates toxins from the system. The formula includes: Citrus Peel, Pinellia, Ma Huang, Fritilliaria, Bamboo Sap, Bupleurum, Hoelen, Platycodon, Xingren, Morus, Magnolia,

Tussilago, Ophiopogon, Schzandra, Ginger, Licorice.

#2. These two combinations are very beneficial for the respiratory system. Fenugreek and Thyme are especially beneficial for the sinuses and head area. They both help prevent and eliminate mucus from the respiratory system. It helps keep the lungs and the nasal passages clean to prevent germs and viruses from multiplying. The formula includes: Fenugreek, Thyme, Marshmallow, Fenugreek, Slippery Elm.

#3. This formula is designed for the nervous and muscle system as well as the respiratory. This supplies nutrients to heal and strengthen the respiratory system. The formula includes: Blessed Thistle, Pleurisy, Skullcap, Yerba Santa.

#4. This formula is excellent for the lungs. It supplies nutrition for the respiratory system. This helps in asthma, allergies, coughs, sinus headache and sinus irritation that causes drainage in the throat. The formula includes: Marshmallow, Chinese Ephedra, Mullein, Passionflower, Catnip, Senega, Slippery Elm.

#5. This formula is designed for the entire respiratory system and is especially effective for the sinuses. It helps clean and strengthen the mucous membranes of the nose, throat and lungs to prevent allergies and other respiratory problems. It helps with hay fever, sinus irritations, itching eyes, irritating coughs, asthma, bronchitis and respiratory infections. The formula includes: Chinese Ephedra, Senega, Goldenseal, Capsicum, Parsley, Chaparral, Burdock.

## SINGLE HERBS FOR THE RESPIRATORY SYSTEM

Angelica, Boneset, Comfrey, Ephedra, Fenugreek, Flaxseed, Goldenseal, Licorice, Lobelia, Marshmallow, Mullein, Yerba Santa

# THE STRUCTURAL SYSTEM

The structural system consists of bones, muscles and connective tissue. Poor nutrition and the inability to assimilate minerals contribute to bone loss. High protein and sugar diets, smoking, alcohol, caffeine drinks, and lack of exercise all contribute to bone loss and pave the way for other diseases.

Bone loss in women after menopause is a special concern. This hapens when decreased secretion of the hormone estrogen is greatest. This isn't necessary if a balanced diet is followed with ample supply of minerals. The ability to assimilate minerals is a concern seen in the young as well as the elderly.

## STRUCTURAL FORMULA

This formula is designed to provide nutrition for the bones, flesh and cartilage of the structural system. There are many nutrients that contribute to a healthy structural system, and the following have been beneficial. The formula includes: vitamin A (beta carotene), vitamin C, calcium (chelated for easier assimilation), iron, vitamins D, B6, B12, Phosphorus, Magnesium, Manganese, Potassium, Horsetail, Betaine HCI (necessary for the assimilation of calcium and other minerals), Papaya, Parsley, Pineapple, Valerian, Licorice, Ma Huang.

## SPECIAL STRUCTURAL FORMULAS

#1. This formula strengthens the structural, nervous and immune systems. This helps prevent arthritis, gout and rheumatism as well as other related problems. The formula includes: Bromelain, Hydrangea, Yucca, Horsetail, Chaparral, Alfalfa, Black Cohosh, Catnip, Yarrow, Capsicum, Valerian, White Willow, Burdock, Slippery Elm, Sarsaparilla.

#2. This is especially beneficial for increasing bone mass as well as strengthening the nervous system. It is rich in calcium as well as minerals to help in the assimilation of calcium. The formula includes: Alfalfa, Marshmallow, Plantain, Horsetail, Oatstraw, Wheat Grass, Hops.

#3. This is formulated to nourish the hair, skin and nails. It is a benefit to the structural system. It is rich in silicon, which has shown to be beneficial to calcium assimilation to strengthen the bones and the entire body. The formula includes: Dulse, Horsetail, Sage, Rosemary.

#4. This is a formula to use internally and externally. It will heal and rebuild tissues. It will help in cases of adhesion, which cause a lot of pain and misery. The formula includes: Slippery Elm, Marshmallow, Goldenseal, Fenugreek.

#5. This Chinese Formula is designed to strengthen the bones. It also helps enhance the urinary system. It helps in backaches, fatigue, arthritis, osteoporosis and tones up the structural system. The formula includes: Eucommia, Cistanche, Rehmannia, Morinda, Drynaria, Achyranthes, Hoelen, Dipsacus, Lycium, Dioscorea, Ligustrum, cornus, Dang Gui (Dong Quai), Panax Ginseng, Astragalus, Epimedium, Liguidambar, Atractylodes.

## SINGLE HERBS FOR THE STRUCTURAL SYSTEM

Aloe Vera, Bayberry, Comfrey, Horsetail, Oatstraw, Red Raspberry, White Oak Bark, Yucca.

# THE URINARY SYSTEM

The urinary system consists of the kidneys, bladder, ureter and urethra. Keeping this system in good working condition will help prevent the body from poisoning itself. The proper function of this system is vital to our inner health. The kidneys help maintain a balance of body fluids. The kidneys have the ability to filter out harmful toxic material while retaining the vital vitamins, proteins, sugars, fats and minerals. But if this system is overloaded with more toxins than it can eliminate, diseases will invade the body. It will cause protein in the blood to be lost in the urine. Potassium, calcium, magnesium and zinc can also be lost. This causes nutritional depletion and illness. Diseases associated with kidney failure are high blood pressure, stroke, heart attack or heart disease. It is important to protect the urinary system and nourish it with the proper food, vitamins, minerals, herbs and supplements that strengthen these vital organs.

## URINARY FORMULA

The following nutrients strengthen the urinary system and prevent kidney and bladder problems. Contains vitamins B1, B2, C, D, Folic acid, Magnesium, Niacinamide, Pantothenic Acid, Potassium, Uva Ursi, Hydrangea, Parsley, Dandelion, Siberian Ginseng, Schizandra, Dong Quai, Cornsilk, Horsetail, Hops, Lemon Bioflavonoids

## SPECIAL URINARY FORMULAS

#1. This formula contains potassium and other essential minerals that are vital for urinary health. The formula includes: Kelp, Dulse, Watercress, Wild Cabbage, Horseradish, Horsetail.

#2. This formula strengthens the urinary, reproductive, and digestive systems. The formula includes: Dong Quai, Goldenseal, Juniper, Uva Ursi, Parsley, Ginger, Marshmallow.

#3. This formula provides nutrition for the urinary system. It will help protect the urinary organs from kidney stones, infections and water retention. The formula includes: Juniper Berries, Parsley, Uva Ursi, Dandelion, Chamomile.

#4. This formula strengthens the urinary system as well as the lymph system. This Chinese formula contains the following: Stephania, Hoelen, Morus, Chaenomeles, Astragalus, Atryctylodes, Alisma, Magnolia, Polyporus, Areca, Aakebia, Cinnamon, Pinellis, Ginger, Citrus Peel, Licorice.

## SINGLE HERBS FOR THE URINARY SYSTEM

Cornsilk, Garlic, Grapevine, Horsetail, Hydrangea, Juniper Berries, Marshmallow, Parsley, Peach Bark, Slippery Elm, Uva Ursi

# Appendix

## HERBAL EXTRACT FORMULAS

In this section I have put together some specific extract formulas and what they are good for. The advantage of extracts is that they either go directly into the bloodstream or are absorbed within minutes in the walls of the stomach. In an extract, the more active principals of medicinal herbs are liberated from insoluble, pulpy material. This is beneficial when digestion is poor, which is usually the problem when one is ill.

There are herbs that extract better in alcohol because it draws out more medicinal properties than vinegar. But vinegar and glycerin are also beneficial ways of extracting herbs. Vegetable glycerin has a sweet taste and is useful for children's remedies. It is a preservative and draws out medicinal properties better than water, but not as well as alcohol. Extracts are excellent to use internally and externally. If using alcohol extracts is a problem, place the amount of extract you will use in a cup of boiling water, allow the alcohol to evaporate, then drink the water.

BONESET, FENUGREEK, HORSERADISH, MULLEIN AND FENNEL
This extract formula is excellent for the lungs. It is soothing, cleansing and healing for the mucous membranes. It helps with

allergies, asthma, bronchitis, emphysema, coughs, congestion, lung ailments, mucus congestion, pneumonia, the immune system and is excellent to help heal and clean the stomach and aid in digestive problems.

## BLACK WALNUT EXTRACT

Black walnut is rich in organic iodine and tannins, both of which contain antiseptic properties. This extract is useful for skin problems, parasites and worms, bruises, itching skin, ringworm, syphilis, and athlete's foot. It can help regulate blood sugar levels and eliminate toxins and fatty material.

## BLUE VERVAIN EXTRACT

This extract is used as a natural tranquilizer because it relaxes the body. It is good for fevers, upset stomach, colds, respiratory problems, spleen and liver conditions. It helps to stimulate suppressed menstruation. This extract is also effective for hysteria, epilepsy, palsy, nervous exhaustion, hallucinations, coughs, earaches, headaches, diarrhea, insomnia and dysentery..

## CAPSICUM EXTRACT

Capsicum is one of the best stimulants in the herbal kingdom. It is healing for the arteries, veins and capillaries. It can help stop bleeding internally and externally. It has been used to stop heart attacks, strokes, colds, flu, low vitality, headaches, indigestion, depression, arthritis and ulcers. This is a good extract to have on hand for emergencies.

## CATNIP AND FENNEL EXTRACT

This is an excellent extract for infants and children. It is relaxing for fevers and restlessness. It can help relieve colic, ease stomach cramps, soothe an upset stomach, reduce acid indigestion and relieve gas. It can be taken internally or simply rubbed on the stomach.

## GARLIC OIL EXTRACT

Garlic is nature's natural antibiotic. This extract is useful for high blood pressure, infections, and earaches. It works well with mullein oil for ear infections.

## ECHINACEA AND GOLDENSEAL EXTRACT

An excellent extract for fighting infections. It acts as a natural antibiotic is good for viral and bacterial infections. It helps with colds, flu, bronchitis, sinus infections, throat problems and coughs. It is effective for cleaning the lymphatic and glandular systems of toxins and mucus.

## GOLDENSEAL AND PARTHENIUM EXTRACT

This extract is useful for infections of all kinds. It can kill parasites and worms and is good to take when traveling to prevent diarrhea. It can help the body heal lymphatic congestion, contagious diseases, childhood diseases, colds, flu and sore throats.

## HAWTHORN BERRY EXTRACT

This extract is beneficial for the circulatory system. It nourishes the heart and can help prevent arteriosclerosis, weak heart action, and angina pectoris. It can heal heart valve defects, an enlarged heart, and breathing problems due to weak heart action and lack of oxygen.

## LICORICE ROOT EXTRACT

Licorice is considered food for the adrenal glands. It stimulates the body to produce interferon, which is an immune substance that counteracts cancer and viruses. It stimulates the body to produce its own natural estrogen and cortisone, an action which helps balance female hormones. This extract is useful for lung conditions, hypoglycemia, diabetes and to help counteract stress. It can also help with hoarseness and throat damage.

## LOBELIA EXTRACT

Lobelia is one of the best relaxants in the herbal kingdom. It is excellent for strengthening the nervous system and cleaning obstruction from the stomach. It helps remove congestion from any part of the body. Lobelia extract is helpful for bronchial spasms, the clearing of allergies, asthma, bronchitis, childhood diseases, convulsions, croup, headaches and spasms. It can be rubbed on a child's spine to promote relaxation and healing.

## GINKGO, KOREA GINSENG AND GOTU KOLA EXTRACT

This herbal extract is excellent for the brain. It can help improve concentration, and memory, as well as reduce the symptons of Alzheimer's and ADD. It helps improve blood circulation so it works to feed, nourish, and clean the brain.

## OREGON GRAPE EXTRACT

This extract works on the liver, blood, stomach and intestines. It helps the body in chronic diseases such as blood poisoning, skin problems, liver congestion, and staph infections. It helps the body heal itself.

## PAU D'ARCO EXTRACT

Pau d'Arco is a natural blood cleanser and builder, and it helps protect the liver from damage. This extract has antibiotic properties which can help destroy viral infections. It has helped in many kinds of cancers. It has been used for healing arthritis, asthma, diabetes, gonorrhea, hernia, infections, liver ailments, lupus, Parkinson's disease, tumors, Epstein-Barr, pyorrhea, skin problems, spleen, ulcers, and varicose veins.

## RED CLOVER, BURDOCK AND SPICE EXTRACT

This is an excellent and proven formula for cleansing the blood and eliminating toxins from the bloodstream. It helps with infections, cancers, skin problems, and chronic diseases. It is a tonic for nerves and is useful for colds, flu and childhood diseases.

### RED RASPBERRY, PEPPERMINT, ROSE HIPS AND HIBISCUS

This is an excellent extract formula for all female problems. It can help reduce nausea during pregnancy and also feeds and strengthens the uterus. It can help in balancing hormones, preventing hemorrhage, reducing pain and curing diarrhea. It is also helpful for children with fevers, colds, colic and vomiting.

### CHAMOMILE, PASSIONFLOWER, FENNEL, MARSHMALLOW, HOPS, AND FEVERFEW EXTRACT

This extract is useful for nervous disorders. It can help the body handle stressful situations by calming for the nerves, relaxing the body and promoting sleep. It is a good remedy for insomnia, irritability and nervous fatigue.

### MA HUANG, WHITE WILLOW, DANDELION, AND STINGING NETTLE EXTRACT

This extract formula increases thermogenesis. It helps to decrease appetite and increase energy levels, so is a good stimulant for weight loss.

### VALERIAN, ANISE, BLACK WALNUT, DESERT TEA, GINGER AND LICORICE EXTRACT

This extract formula contains antispasmodic properties to strengthen the nervous system. It helps repair and rebuild the nervous system. It helps with spastic conditions, convulsions, asthma attacks, nervous disorders, insomnia and fevers. It is an excellent formula for acute and chronic diseases.

### DANDELION, INDIGO, THLASPI, BUPLEURUM, SCUTE, PINELLIA, GINSENG, CINNAMON AND LICORICE EXTRACT

This extract is formulated to strengthen and provide nutritional support to the immune system. It can help improve the digestive system and the liver. This formula can help in healing the many autoimmune disease that are plaguing mankind.

# COMMON POULTICES

*Bayberry:* Can be applied to skin for cancerous and ulcerated sores. It is a strong cleanser and healer.

*Catnip:* Reduces swelling, especially good for under the eyes. Culpeper mentions catnip for hemorrhoids, applied topically.

*Clay:* Excellent healing agent. Good for skin problems such as eczema. Swollen liver can be helped with clay packs. It is suggested that clay should be taken internally a few days before using it as a pack on the body. It can be used for boils, carbuncles and tumors.

*Comfrey:* Excellent for healing wounds and broken bones. It can be applied externally for burns, sprains and wounds and has been used as a hot poultice to help ease pain caused by bursitis.

*Ginger:* Add powdered ginger to boiling water. Soak a cloth in ginger water and apply to affected areas to help relieve pain, or to bring blood to the surface of congested areas. Ginger baths and soaking the feet will help reduce pain.

*Hops:* A poultice made of hops soothes inflammations and boils and helps reduce the pain of toothache. Its lupulon and humulon properties help to prevent infections.

*Mullein:* Used for swollen lymph glands and lymph congestion. Use one part lobelia and three parts mullein.

*Onion:* Used for boils, ears, infections, sore throats, and sores. When using as a poultice, chop and heat the onions.

*Plantain:* This is a valuable first-aid remedy. Apply mashed or crushed herb on a cut, swollen or running sore and secure with a clean bandage. Discard pulp and replace as needed.

*Potato:* Good for infections, tumors and warts. Use by grating raw potato and add ginger (to stimulate the action of the potato).

*Slippery Elm:* Excellent for abscesses, bites, blood poison, boils, and stings. (Note: Slippery elm is used as a jelling agent for poultices. It is excellent mixed with other herbs.)

*White Oak Bark:* Use for hemorrhoids and varicose veins.

*Yarrow:* This is a good poultice for wounds and inflammations. It has been used to reduce swellings and ease earaches. The poultice will also soothe bruises and abrasions. For nosebleeds, the leaves are steeped in water and then placed in the nostrils. It is also useful for nicks and cuts. Yarrow has anti-inflammatory properties and can be applied as a tea to sore nipples in nursing mothers. It can be used as a wash for eczema, rashes, and poison ivy.

# NATURAL ANTISEPTICS

*Black Walnut:* external and internal antiseptic, good for internal parasites, infection and tonsillitis.

*Cabbage Leaves:* contains rapine, an antibiotic. The warm leaves placed on the ulcerated sore will draw out the pus on sores.

*Carrots:* mashed and boiled and applied to a sore have helped in drawing out pus and healing the area. It is said to be a strong antiseptic.

*Clove:* the oil is strong germicide. It is used for toothaches, and pains as well as nausea and vomiting.

*Cornflowers:* contain important glycosides which have strong antiseptic properties. This herb has been used in eyewashes. Its antigermicidal and antibacterial properties have been used as an effective antidote against snake venom and scorpion poisons.

*False Unicorn:* contains chamaelirin, a strong antiseptic. Helps ease evacuation of tapeworms and worms in the intestinal tract. It creates a healthful pure environment in the body.

*Garlic:* is a powerful antibacterial agent. It contains allicin. The powder on wounds is good for the healing process. Garlic oil is useful for ear infections.

*Goldenseal:* contains the antibiotic berberine which is used for mouth/gum problems. It is also used for worms and infection.

*Lemons:* a natural antiseptic. Helps fade freckles.

*Myrrh:* has sensational antiseptic properties, contains gums, essential oils, resins and other bitter compounds. Good for uterus and vaginal infections and dysentery. It is also used for serious periodontal diseases. Laboratory tests have proven this to be one of the finest antibacterial and antiviral agents.

*Tea Tree Oil:* Contains antifungal properties. It aids with conditions such as athlete's foot, acne, boils, burns, warts, vaginal infections, tonsillitis, sinus infections, ringworm, skin rashes, impetigo, herpes, corns, head lice, cold sores, canker sores, insect bites and fungal infections. It is a remarkable oil with valuable properties for healing.

*Thyme:* contains an antiseptic called thymol. Use small amounts for dressing wounds. Thyme should be crushed and added to boiling water, then steeped and strained. It can be used for sprains and bruises.

*Queen of the Meadow:* used as an antiseptic to treat diseases of the uterus and cancer of the womb.

# EMERGENCY AIDS

## ALCOHOLISM

*Hops:* good for delirium

*Cayenne:* reduces dilated blood vessels

*Goldenseal:* natural antibiotic

*Chaparral:* helps clean the residue of alcohol

*Bee Pollen:* gives nourishment and strength to the body

*Glutamine (amino acid):* has been used in large doses to reduce the craving for alcohol

## ALLERGIES

The best natural antihistamine is to cut orange peels in small strips and soak in apple cider vinegar for several hours, drain and cook down in honey until soft (but not the consistency of candy). Keep in refrigerator and use as needed. Relieves stuffiness and clogged passages. Allergies are treated with tyrosine, especially cases of hayfever from grass pollen.

## ARTHRITIS

*Histidine:* is good for tissue growth and repair and is useful for its anti-inflammatory effect and is used in rheumatoid arthritis.

*Proline (amino acid):* is used in multiple amino acid and vitamin formula for arthritis

## ASTHMA

For an acute attack, a few drops of lobelia extract in the mouth will relax and put a stop to the spasms. Pour one cup cold water over one or two teaspoons of shredded elecampane root. Let stand eight to ten hours, then reheat. Take very hot, in small sips. Can sweeten with honey. Use one cup twice a day.

## BLEEDING

*Cayenne pepper:* a small amount applied in the nose has stopped bleeding immediately, taken internally with water helps internal bleeding, also helps a bleeding cut

*Plantain:* powdered herb or fresh leaf applied directly on wound, dampen first

*Marigold:* the tincture in boiled water used to wash wounds, very useful in bleeding conditions

*Shepherd's Purse:* works as a styptic. Use as a tea and apply as a poultice to the wound

## BLISTERS

The amino acid methionine helps heal rashes and blisters in babies with high ammonia content in their urine. The amino acid Lysine has helped heal fever blisters when given 500 milligrams of lysine daily, with acidophilus and yogurt.

## BOILS

*Figs:* fresh figs applied hot, also used for mouth sores

*Honey:* an antibiotic, apply with a small amount of comfrey powder, apply and it will help bring boils to a head

*Slippery elm:* use the powder added to water to make a paste, healing as a poultice, can be used for wounds, boils and skin problems

## BRONCHITIS

*Comfrey, Mullein, and Lobelia:* are excellent for bronchitis. Bowels must be opened, an enema is helpful.

*Lobelia tincture:* for immediate needs if there is shortness of breath or gasping, if the throat needs to be cleared of mucus, a few drops of lobelia tincture will relax the throat and bronchi

*Irish moss:* good for chronic bronchitis

*Cysteine (amino acid):* has the ability to build white cell activity and helps build resistance for respiratory diseases such as chronic bronchitis, emphysema, and and tuberculosis

## BRUISES

*Comfrey powder, goldenseal mixed with aloe vera juice* is very good for bruises.

*Mullein:* oil of mullein flowers with olive oil is good for bruises

*St. John's wort:* the flowers are infused in olive oil and applied to bruises and wounds

*Shepherd's purse:* the whole plant as a poultice for wounds

*Witch Hazel:* a compress dipped in distilled witch hazel is good for bruises and swellings

## BURNS

*Immediately immerse* in cool water, apply vitamin E oil and take vitamin E orally

*Aloe vera plant:* cut off leaves, slit them open and squeeze juice onto burn, or lay exposed side of leaf directly on burn

*Wheat germ oil and honey:* make a paste of wheat germ oil and honey in blender, mixing at low speed, then add comfrey leaves to make a thick paste. Apply to burn and keep remainder in refrigerator.

*Marshmallow compress:* can be used for mild burns

*Potatoes:* peeled raw potatoes will help on burns

*Vitamin C:* applied topically and taken internally reduces pain eliminating the need for morphine

## CHAPPED HANDS

*Aloe vera gel* can be applied to chapped hands and chapped lips

## CHICKEN POX

*External teas:* red raspberry, catnip, peppermint with vinegar to relieve itching

*Goldenseal tea:* for severe itching

*Lemonade* with honey andfresh vegetable and fruit juices, if possible

## COLDS AND FLU

*Use mild teas* made from catnip or peppermint or red raspberry, use boneset, elderberry and peppermint teas for cases of the flu, give natural vitamin C liquid.

*Chamomile tea:* relaxing and soothing for colds and flu

*Lemon and honey water:* steeped and used for colds and coughs, refreshing and restorative

*Honey:* added to herb drinks will help destroy bacteria for the honey is a bactericide

*Barley water:* wash two ounces of barley and boil in one pint of water for a few minutes. Discard water then place barley in four pints pure water. Add clean lemon peel and boil down to two pints. Strain and add two ounces of honey. Can be used freely for children.

## CONSTIPATION

Prevention is the best method. The diet for children should include whole-grain cereals, leafy greens, and raw fruits with skins. These are essential in keeping the bowels working normally. Emotional disturbances in the mother affect the baby if nursing.

*Chamomile tea:* weak chamomile tea is good for constipation
*Cascara Sagrada:* small amounts for children.
*Elderflower:* good in cases of constipation
*Licorice:* added to herbal teas has a slight laxative action

## CONVULSIONS

*Weak chamomile tea* in small doses several times a day helps. A warm chamomile tea enema is helpful.
*Lobelia tincture* can also be rubbed well into the neck, chest and between the shoulder.

## COUGHS

*Onion remedy:* peel, and chop onions, cover with honey. Simmer. Strain and use as a cough syrup.
*Honey and licorice root* or honey and horehound herb, or honey and wild cherry bark are useful
*Mullein:* good for croup cough
*Combination* of marshmallow, mullein, comfrey, lobelia and chickweed in equal parts are good for coughs
*Pitted dates* crushed and made into a syrup has been used for coughs, sore throat and bronchitis
*Tea of sage and thyme* in equal parts with a pinch of cardamon and ginger and cloves and nutmeg is another remedy for coughs

## HEAVY COUGH

*Cherry bark and coltsfoot tea:* chew on licorice or candied ginger
*Almond drink:* For cough and fever, grind almonds into powder and steep in one pint cold water

*Horehound remedy:* use two tablespoons of the fresh leaves with two cups of boiling water, drink in small amounts

## CROUP

*Catnip or chamomile tea:* bring perspiration

*A few drops of lobelia tincture* in catnip or peppermint tea is helpful.

## DEPRESSION

*Tyrosine* has been found to have a fantastic effect on depression for its management and control and compared to a drug used for depression with one great difference—no side effects.

*Gotu Kola:* helps in mental fatigue which is common in depression.

*Ginseng:* helps stimulate the entire body energy to overcome depression

*Kelp:* contains all the minerals for glandular health

*Herbal combinations:* Black cohosh, capsicum, valerian, mistletoe, ginger, St. John's wort, hops, wood betony

## DIARRHEA

*Red Raspberry tea* is soothing for diarrhea

*Carob Powder* in boiled milk—usually about one teaspoon to one cup milk.

*Barley water* given to small babies is good for diarrhea.

*Licorice or Ginger* is good to help colic pains from diarrhea

*Carrot soup:* is an excellent remedy for infant diarrhea, the cooked soup coats the inflamed small bowel, soothes it, and helps promote healing.

*Slippery Elm Tea:* nourishing as well as healing

*Ginger:* a weak ginger tea settles the stomach and helps in diarrhea.

## DIPHTHERIA

*Pineapple juice,* lemon juice and honey or cider vinegar and honey is useful.

*A pinch of cayenne* can be used for older children

## EARACHE

*Oil of garlic in the ear:* hold in with cotton
*Oil of lobelia in each ear:* hold in with cotton

## FEVER

*High fevers:* an enema is needed to reduce the temperature.
*Barley water for high fever:* (use linen cloth to tie barley and boil for
    1/2 hour)

## HEADACHES

*Capsuled Hops with water*
*Wood betony, Chamomile tea, Tei-Fu Oil* rubbed on temples.
*For severe headaches:* fasting with juice and green drinks.

## HEMORRHOIDS

*Ginger tea,* yarrow extract, white oak bark. Applied externally.

## HERPES SIMPLEX I (*FEVER BLISTERS OR COLD SORES*)

*Lysine* inhibits the virus, together with vitamin C, A and zinc.
*Yogurt and buttermilk* will eliminate the pain, halt the spread of the
    lesions and promote healing

## HERPES SIMPLEX II

*Black walnut:* used internally as well as externally
*Goldenseal:* mixed with aloe vera for external use, internally to
    speed healing of infection.

## INSECT BITES AND BEE STINGS

*Clay:* a clay paste dampened and applied to the bite and sting will
    help relieve the pain
*Plantain:* wet plantain leaf with a little olive oil and place on bee or
    hornet sting, after the stinger is removed will help to heal, you
    need to replace the leaf as it dries.
*Honey:* apply honey after removing the stinger
*Comfrey:* mixed with aloe vera juice will reduce swelling

## INSOMNIA

*Plain, warm milk* contains generous amounts of the amino acid Tryptophan which quiets the nervous system and when taken with vitamin B6 keeps the Tryptophan high in the blood stream. It is an essential ingredient for the regeneration of the body tissues. This is a natural alternative to tranquilizers.

*Hops:* help relax the body

*Herbal calcium* combinations helps

*Passionflower:* excellent for insomnia

*Valerian:* can be used occasionally, prolonged use can cause depression in some people

## KIDNEY STONES

*Apple juice and lemon juice fasts* with olive oil.

## MEASLES

*Hot catnip tea* or chamomile tea will break out the rash and check the fever, three tablespoons of the herb in a quart of water and boiled down to one pint.

## MEMORY

*Glutamine* has been used with safety when given to children who can't learn or retain information.

*Gotu Kola* has been used with children to improve their learning ability and concentration

## MUMPS

*Hot catnip tea* relieves pain.

## RINGWORM

*A fungoid parasite* is best stopped by sealing off the air.

*Undiluted lemon juice, white of egg, nail varnish:* apply every few hours

*Garlic:* used internally is helpful

*Apply tincture* of lobelia and olive oil

## SUNBURN

*To avoid sunburn* mix one teaspoon vinegar to 1/2 cup thin sunflower oil and apply.

*Gel from aloe vera* plant is useful for sunburn

*Equal parts of honey and wheat germ oil* with powdered comfrey added. Make paste ahead and it will keep well in a covered jar.

## TOOTHACHE

*Hot poultices* will reduce the pain of toothache

*Chamomile and hop tea* will help relax the body

*Oil of clove:* clove oil can be mixed with zinc oxide powder to form a paste, this will protect the cavity from food

## TONSILLITIS

*Catnip tea enema:* pineapple juice

*Vegetable juices* are useful in removing waste

*Red raspberry tea:* comfrey tea

## WEIGHT CONTROL

*Phenylalanine:* is effective in weight control because of its positive effect on the thyroid.

*Kelp:* helps regulate the thyroid

*Fasting Formula:* Licorice, Beet Root, Hawthorne and Fennel

## WORMS

*Grated raw apples* sprinkled with anise seed in a salad will get rid of worms

*Cold sage tea* is also good for worms

*Garlic:* Excellent body cleanser

*Papaya Latex* is used in Asia for children to expel worms (obtain at health food stores)

*Yarrow:* tonic to the bowels after expelling worms

*Pomegranate:* good for pin worms, round worms and tape worms

*Pumpkin seeds:* help eliminate worms

# HERBAL FIRST AID KIT

The following list comprises herbs and other medicinal items that could come in handy if regularly kept in a first aid kit.

*Aloe Vera Gel:* Excellent for burns and skin rashes, also used for insect bites and stings, poison oak and ivy, acne and itchy skin.

*Antispasmodic Extract:* contains valerian, anise, lobelia, black walnut, brigham tea, licorice and ginger. Used for the nerves and spastic conditions, excellent in emergency conditions such as hysteria, shock, poisonous bites and stings, used externally for pain and muscular spasms.

*Capsicum:* Powder and extract, can be rubbed on toothaches, inflammation and swellings, in treating arthritis, rub capsicum extract over the inflamed joint and wrap with flannel for the night. Is useful to stop bleeding internally and externally by helping to normalize the circulation. Capsicum and plantain will draw out foreign bodies embedded in the skin.

*Cascara Sagrada:* safe tonic, laxative, very important to keep the bowels open in illness and avoid constipation.

*Chamomile:* used as a tea, is safe for children in colds, indigestion and nervous disorders, relieves menstrual cramps, externally, apply to swellings, sore muscles and painful joints.

*Charcoal:* used for diarrhea and intestinal gas, can be used as a poultice. Can be used in some poisoning.

*Chlorophyll:* I keep liquid chlorophyll on hand for all kinds of emergencies. It is a good cleanser for the blood. It is good to clean the bowels. Good for children and nursing mothers. It is rich in minerals.

*Comfrey:* Can be used for bleeding by using a strong decoction. It can be used internally and externally for healing of fractures, wounds, sores and ulcers. It is an old time remedy from the Middle Ages, and is as follows: place burned area in ice water until pain is gone; mix the following in blender—1/2 cup wheat germ oil, 1/2 cup honey, and add as much dried or fresh comfrey leaves as it will take to make a thick paste and add a pinch of lobelia.

*Eucalyptus Oil:* useful for bronchial spasms, chills, colds, sore throat, rheumatism, good antiseptic and expectorant.

*Flowers And Plants, Edible And Nutritious:* Chicory, Clover, Dandelion, Elderberry, Squash, Borage, Nasturtium Lamb's Quarters, Plaintain, Purslane, Rose Petals Violets and Wild Watercress.

*Fenugreek:* dissolves mucus, good for infections of nose, throat and lungs. Helps to lower fevers. Excellent for children.

*Garlic powder and oil:* "Nature's antibiotic", the oil is used for ear aches. Garlic taken with capsicum and vitamin C at the beginning of a cold will often help.

*Ginger:* excellent for upset stomach, nausea, colds and flu.

*Lobelia Extract:* can be used internally and externally to relax all spasms, a few drops in the ear will relieve earaches, lobelia used with catnip as an enema is effective for fevers and infections, used externally in baths, compressions, poultices, and liniments for muscle spasms.

*Peppermint Oil:* Aids nausea, an excellent stomach aid, assists in digestion, cleanses and gives tone to the entire body, sedative for nervous and restless persons of all ages, promotes relaxation and sleep.

*Red Raspberry:* excellent for pregnancy, relieving nausea, prevents hemorrhage, reduces pain and eases childbirth, reliable for children for stomach problems, fevers, colds and flu.

*Sarsaparilla:* a hot decoction, made with an ounce of root in a pint of water, will promote profuse sweating and will act as a powerful agent to expel gas from the stomach and intestines.

*Tea tree oil:* contains antifungal properties, and helps with conditions such as athlete's foot, acne, boils, burns, warts, vaginal infections, tonsillitis, sinus infections, ringworm, skin rashes, impetigo, herpes, corns, head lice, cold sores, canker sores, insect bites and fungal infections.

# Bibliography

Airola, Paavo, Ph.D., N.D.
HOW TO GET WELL
Health Plus, publisher, 1974

Bethel, May
THE HEALING POWER OF HERBS, 1969
THE HEALING POWER OF NATURAL FOODS, 1978

Bianchini, Francesco, and Corbetta, Francesco
HEALTH PLANTS OF THE WORLD
Newsweek Books, New York

Bircher, Benner, M., M.D.
THE BIRCHER: BENNER CHILDRENS DIET BOOK
Keats Publishing, Inc. 1977
New Cannan, Connecticut

Castleman, Michael
THE HEALING HERBS
Rodale, 1991
Emmaus, Pennsylvania

Challen, Jack Joseph and Renate Lewin
WHAT HERBS ARE ALL ABOUT
Keats Publishing, Inc, 1980

Christopher, Dr. John R.
THE SCHOOL OF NATURAL HEALING
BiWorld Publishers 1976
Clymer, R. Swinburne, M.D.
NATURE'S HEALING AGENTS
The Humanitarian Society, First Printing 1905

Colby, Benjamin
GUIDE TO HEALTH, 1846 reprint
BiWorld Publishers, Orem, Utah

Coon, Nelson
USING PLANTS FOR HEALING
Hearthside Press 1963
Rodale Press 1979

Culpeper, Nicholas
CULPEPPER'S' HERBAL REMEDIES
Melvin Powers Wilshire Book Co., 1971
CULPEPPER'S COMPLETE HERBAL
W. Foulshan and Co., Ltd.

Dawson, Adele G.
HEALTH, HAPPINESS AND THE PURSUIT OF HERBS
The Stephen Greene Press, Vermont, 1980

Destreot, Raymond
OUR EARTH, OUR CURE
Swan House Publishing Co, 1974

Farwell, Edith Foster
A BOOK OF HERBS
The White Pine Press, 1979

Fluck, Professor Hans
MEDICINAL PLANTS
Translated from German by Rowson, J. M.
W. Foulsham & Co., Ltd, England 1973

Gerard, John
THE HERBAL: THE COMPLETE 1633 EDITION
Revised and enlarged by Thomas Johnson
Dover Publications, Inc. New York 1975

Gibbons, Euell
STALKING THE WILD ASPARAGUS
David McKay Co., Inc. New York 1962

Graedon, Joe
THE PEOPLE'S PHARMACY
Avon Publishers,New York 1980

Grieve, M.
A MODERN HERBAL, Two Volumes
Dover Publications, Inc.

Griffin, LaDean
IS ANY SICK AMONG YOU?
BiWorld Publishers, 1974

Harris, Ben Charles
THE COMPLETE HERBAL
Larchmont Books, New York, 1972

EAT THE WEEDS
Keats Publishing, Inc., 1961

Hutchens, Alma R.
INDIAN HERBOLOGY OF NORTH AMERICA
Merco, 1973

Jensen, Dr. Bernard D. C.
NATURE HAS A REMEDY, 1978

Kadans, Joseph, N. D., Phd.
ENCYCLOPEDIA OF MEDICINAL HERBS
Arco Publishing, Inc. New York 1970

ENCYCLOPEDIA OF FRUITS, VEGETABLES, NUTS AND
SEEDS FOR HEALTHFUL LIVING

Kirschmann, John D. Director
NUTRITION ALMANAC, Revised Edition
McGraw Hill, 1979

Kloss, Jethro
BACK TO EDEN
Published and Distributed by the Jethro Kloss Family
Loma Linda, Ca.

Kordel, Lelord
NATURAL FOLD REMEDIES
Manor Books, Inc. 1974

Krochmal, Arnold and Connie
A GUIDE TO THE MEDICINAL PLANTS OF THE UNITED STATES
The New York Times Book Co. 1973

Kroeger, Hanna
GOOD HEALTH THROUGH DIETS
Boulder, Colorado

Lewis, Walter H. and Memory P. F. Elvin,
MEDICAL BOTANY: PLANTS OF THE UNITED STATES
The New York Times Book Co. 1973

Malstrom, Dr. Stan N. D., M. T.
OWN YOUR OWN BODY
Fresh mountain Air Pub. Co. 1977
HERBAL REMEDIES II REVISED
Woodland Books, 1975

McCleod, Dawn
HERB HANDBOOK
Wilshire Book Co. 1968
North Hollywood, Ca.

MERCK MANUAL, 9th Edition
Merck and Co., Inc.

Meyer, Joseph E.
THE HERBALIST
Meyerbooks, 1960

Montagna, F. Joseph
P.D.R.: PEOPLES DESK REFERENCE VOL I AND II
Quest For Truth Publications, Inc.
Lake Oswego, Oregon 1979

Moore, Michael
MEDICINAL PLANTS OF THE MOUNTAIN WEST
The Museum of New Mexico Press, 1980

Murray, Michael, N.D., and Joseph Pizzorno, N.D.
ENCYCLOPEDIA OF NATURAL MEDICINE
Prima Publishing, 1991
Rocklin, California

Murray, Michael, N.D.
THE HEALING POWER OF HERBS
Prima Publishing, 1995
Rocklin, California

Pahlow, Mannfried
LIVING MEDICINE
Thorsons Publishers Ltd.,England, 1980

Rau, Henrietta A. Diers
HEALING WITH HERBS
Arco Publishing, Inc. New York 1976

Schauenberg, Paul and Paris, Ferdinand
GUIDE TO MEDICINAL PLANTS
Keats Publishing, 1977

Shook, Dr. Edward E.
ELEMENTARY TREATISE IN HERBOLOGY: 1974
ADVANCED TREATISE IN HERBOLOGY: 1978
Trinity Center Press

Thomson, William A.R. M.D., Edited by,
MEDICINES FROM THE EARTH
McGraw: Hill Book Co. New York 1978

Tierra, Michael, C.A., N.D.
THE WAY OF HERBS
Unity Press, Santa Cruz, 1980

United States Pharmacopeial Convention
THE PHYSICIANS' AND PHARMACISTS' GUIDE TO YOUR MEDICINES
Ballantine Books: New York, 1981

Vogel, Dr. Alfred
THE NATURE DOCTOR, 1952

Wade, Carlson
BEE POLLEN AND YOUR HEALTH
Keats Publishing, Inc. Conn.1978

NATURAL HORMONES: THE SECRET OF YOUTHFUL HEALTH
Parker Publishing Co., Inc. New York, 1972

Wren, R. C.
POTTER'S NEW CYCLOPEDIA OF MEDICINAL HERBS AND PREPARATIONS
Harper Colophon Books

# Index